THE WELLNESS FOR LIFE WORKBOOK

STRESS MANAGEMENT

PHYSICAL ACTIVITY

NUTRITION

WEIGHT CONTROL

CHEMICAL INDEPENDENCE

Thomas A. Murphy
and
Dianne Murphy

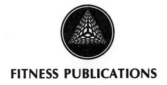

FITNESS PUBLICATIONS

First edition (The Personal Fitness Workbook) 1982
Second edition 1983
Third edition (The Wellness For Life Workbook) 1984
Fourth edition 1987

FITNESS PUBLICATIONS
Hamilton, Montana

ISBN 0-9611482-3-3

TABLE OF CONTENTS

INTRODUCTION

Over time, you are either strengthened or weakened by what you do with yourself on a regular basis. Your present state of wellness and your life-long well-being are largely determined by your accustomed patterns of thought and behavior. The way you eat, your level of physical activity, how you handle stress and your avoidance of chemical dependencies all affect your ability to function effectively, and to enthusiastically partake of the good life. To a large extent, these aspects of your lifestyle determine the mileage you're likely to get out of your natural gifts. They either squander or preserve your basic genetic endowment.

What does it mean to enjoy a high level of wellness? Beyond the absence of illness and pain, wellness means feeling really alive, with a genuine gusto for life, and having plenty of energy to enjoy it fully. It's a trim, flexible, well toned body, a twinkle in your eye, and a warm, friendly smile on your face. In short, wellness is your capacity to live life to its fullest.

On the other hand, over the long term a lack of wellness can lead not only to a loss of trim appearance and vitality, but also to a heightened susceptibility to injury and to many of the major health problems of our time...among them heart and arterial disease, stroke, cancer, diabetes, cirrhosis, emphysema and bronchitis.

Your Wellness For Life program begins with a Lifestyle Inventory which quickly gives you a clear picture of how your current lifestyle patterns are shaping your future well-being. You then receive specific information regarding the various wellness-related lifestyle factors in a concise yet comprehensive statement of the essentials of healthful living. And, as you go on, Wellness For Life introduces you to a completely personalized Living Well program which allows you to gradually build optimal patterns of living into your own way of life, starting from wherever you are right now.

Wellness For Life is designed to enhance virtually every facet of your experience, including your physical, emotional, intellectual and spiritual functioning. As you progress in the Living Well program, you're likely to notice that you're enjoying a greater measure of fulfillment in many important areas: your family life, your social interactions, your professional attainment, as well as your artistic, cultural and recreational pursuits. That's because your capacity for effective performance in every arena is directly supported by your overall level of health and well-being.

And now, enjoy the process of discovering just how easy and fun it really can be to make well-informed decisions today that help to maintain your strength, vitality and productivity for the rest of your life. Take this opportunity to tap the fountain of youth that is hidden within you.

Wellness is a quality of life. It's having the personal energy you need to look and feel well, fulfill your responsibilities, effectively handle emergencies, and actively pursue your social, economic, cultural, spiritual and recreational interests.

No matter who you are or what you do, being well has a positive influence on virtually every aspect of your life—on how you look, how you feel, how you see yourself, and how you perform from day to day.

And over the long haul, a lack of wellness leads to degeneration of critical body functions, greatly increasing the risk of major disease and eventual loss of ability.

Your wellness is a matter of choice

Your wellness is clearly not a matter of right or wrong, good or bad, should or shouldn't. It **is** a matter of making **intelligent choices.** Choices **based upon the best available information** regarding the effects of your behavior on your personal health and well-being. This workbook, therefore, deliberately avoids the implication that you should or should not do anything. Rather, it recognizes your ability to **shape your own lifestyle**; your ability to make choices that reflect your present level of knowledge. By choosing wellness now, you are opening the door to an even more enjoyable and rewarding life in the years yet to come.

Wellness is your heritage

Your body is the product of perhaps 40,000 generations of human development. If you were born into any but the last two or three of these generations, odds are your lifestyle would be far more active than it is now. For the most part, your food would be fresh, close to its naturally grown state. And your survival would depend as much upon your physical prowess as upon your social skills and mental agility. Throughout this formative period, strength, mobility and endurance were essential to the continuance of life, and fitness was an inevitable by-product of being alive.

Not so today. For many people in the modern world, the recent explosive development of complex social systems, agriculture, science and technology has nearly eliminated the physical exertion of work, as well as the threat of immediate food shortages. This affluence presents the new and demanding challenge of maintaining your personal wellness in a culture which makes few physical demands and which presses on all sides with an abundance of over-rich, over-processed foods. You are now presented with a choice of many possible lifestyles, not all of which will assure the maintenance of your personal wellness.

Your wellness is cumulative

The effects of your lifestyle are cumulative, increasingly determining the form, composition and functional effectiveness of your body. In general, the younger you are, the less apparent the effects of your lifestyle will be. As you grow older, your body is slowly shaped by the patterns of your experience, and the physical effects of your lifestyle become more pronounced. The living patterns which keep you well also help you to retain your youthful appearance, vitality and general state of fitness.

A simple formula for success. Your wellness is largely determined by your lifestyle. Simply by exercising properly for 1 hour every other day, eating and drinking well, and not smoking or misusing drugs, you may raise your physical, mental and emotional efficiency 20 to 50 percent, increase your energy production 50 to 200 percent, and greatly reduce your risk of ill health.

The Influence of Lifestyle

Lifestyle is easily the largest single determinant of your overall wellness. This is illustrated by the following breakdown of the influence of the four major factors on death by all causes:

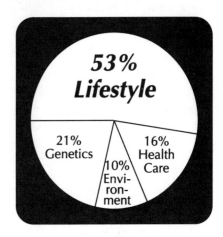

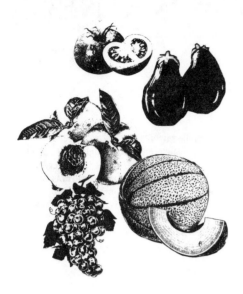

Eat Well!

A lack of wellness is often at the root of common problems such as:

- a lack of energy and vitality
- looking and feeling out of shape
- difficulty coping with daily pressures
- nagging aches and pains
- over- or under-weight
- shortness of breath
- frequent minor illnesses
- loss of muscle tone
- persistent lower back pain
- diminished work performance
- difficulty concentrating
- more frequent emotional upsets
- lowered endurance
- limited flexibility
- greater susceptibility to accidents

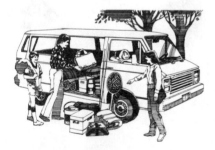

Relax!

Everyone can do it

It doesn't matter how old you are, what shape you're in now, or how long it's been since you were last active. Nearly everyone can be well with surprisingly little effort.

Simply stated, the three basic elements of an effective personal wellness program are:

1. Regularly engage in concentrated physical activity which utilizes the full range of your physical potential.

2. Continually balance your nutritional intake against your current activity level and your changing body composition.

3. Respond to the stresses in your life in potentially fulfilling ways.

Create Your Own Personal Program For Living Well

As you proceed through the Workbook, opportunities are provided for you to set personal objectives in each of the key lifestyle areas. Having selected your goals, you'll be able to monitor your daily living patterns by using the convenient Living Well Daily Performance forms that are provided on pages 60-65. The result is a fully personalized program, created by you, that will allow you to systematically enhance the quality of your lifestyle. This Living Well program is a pleasant wellness game that you can begin playing right now, and continue to enjoy for the rest of your life.

Living Well is a cyclical program, with each cycle lasting six weeks. At the beginning of each six week period, use the Lifestyle Inventory to get a full reading on your present status in all the key wellness categories. With this overview as a point of reference, you're then prepared to select a set of Living Well goals for the upcoming six weeks.

In setting your goals, remember not to overdo it. Just bear in mind that the most important ingredient of Living Well for a lifetime is your eventual success over the long term. Obviously it's far more desirable to achieve gradual mastery over all important factors than it is to become frustrated with a valiant but brief attempt to do everything at once. In any event, you're likely to notice that you're making more healthful choices in all areas, whether or not you've set formal goals for yourself in them at the outset.

Keep Track of Your Daily Living Patterns

In addition to informing yourself about the various factors that are known to affect your wellness, perhaps the most effective step you can take at this time is to begin monitoring your lifestyle patterns in the thirteen key areas discussed throughout the workbook. By continuing to systematically monitor your actual behavior, you'll assure yourself of gradually building an ever increasing measure of well-being into your life.

As you proceed through each section of the Workbook, you'll be introduced to the corresponding portion of the Living Well Daily Performance Record—a tool that you can use to keep track of how well you are doing.

The Wellness For Life Point System

While all the factors that have been included in the Wellness For Life program are supported by extensive research, the relative importance of each individual factor with respect to all others has, in most cases, not been clearly determined.

Consequently the Wellness For Life point system arbitrarily assigns an equal value of 210 points to each of the three general categories of stress management, physical activity and nutrition. Within each of these areas, the minimum number of points obtainable is 70, so an additional 140 points can be earned in each category through the implementation of healthful behaviors.

In the area of Potential Dependencies, the maximum number of points obtainable is 0, and the minimum is 140—that is, up to 140 points can be lost through the abuse of chemicals.

So, for the system as a whole, the maximum number of points obtainable is 630, and the minimum number is 70. Within each category, points are distributed among the various factors in a manner which attempts to recognize their potential contribution to the maintenance of overall good health. In the area of nutrition, for example, you can earn 75 of the 210 total points by eating unrefined carbohydrates, 75 points by controlling your intake of fats, and another 60 points by eating in moderation.

Plan Ahead For Best Results

Use the Living Well Planning Calendar on the following page to smoothly integrate your new lifestyle patterns into your accustomed way of life. You may also find it useful in gaining an overview of the way you are utilizing your time in general.

Begin by taking a look at how your time is now allocated. For example, if you sleep 8 hours a day, and you work 40 hours per week, then you have about 72 hours each week to use in other ways, and your weekly calendar might look something like this:

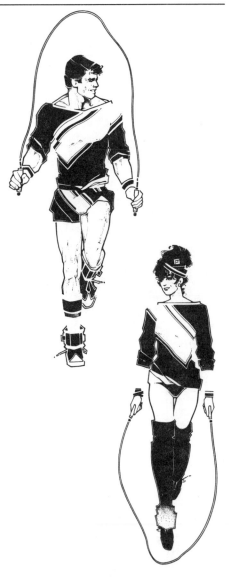

Regularly Engage in Proper Physical Activity!

	SUN	MON	TUE	WED	THU	FRI	SAT
6- 7 AM	J	S,T,B	R	S,T,B	J	S,T,B	S
7- 8							
8- 9		W O R K					
9-10							
10-11							
11-12							
12- 1 PM							
1- 2		W O R K					
2- 3							
3- 4							
4- 5							
5- 6							
6- 7							
7- 8			Class		R		
8- 9			Class				
9-10	C	C	C	C	C	C	C
10-11							
11-12							
12- 1 AM							
1- 2		S L E E P					
2- 3							
3- 4							
4- 5							
5- 6							

KEY:

J   Stretch (5 min), Jog (30 min)
S   Full Body Stretch (15 min)
T   Body Toning (20-30 min)
B   Exercise Bicycle (30 min)
R   Racquetball (60 min)
C   Conscious Relaxation (10 min)

Obviously, this is an example only, and your own calendar may bear little resemblance to this one. The point is that you can arrange your wellness activities in whatever manner is best suited to your needs. The value of time planning is in the expression of your intentions in concrete, practical terms.

3

Wellness Planning Calendar

	SUN	MON	TUE	WED	THU	FRI	SAT
6-7 AM							
7-8							
8-9							
9-10							
10-11							
11-12							
12-1 PM							
1-2							
2-3							
3-4							
4-5							
5-6							
6-7							
7-8							
8-10							
10 PM TO 6 AM							

1. First color in the blocks representing the days and hours that you ordinarily spend at work.
2. Next (perhaps using a different color), fill in the blocks that represent your usual hours of sleep.
3. Then identify any other time periods that you have already committed to regular activities.
4. With this information in hand, you'll be able to identify the best times to accomplish the various Living Well activities as they are presented throughout the Workbook.

HOW YOU SEE YOURSELF

The term "wellness" is of relatively recent vintage. It came into being primarily because the notion of "health" has so often referred simply to an absence of illness. It is easy to see, however, that even in the absence of obvious symptoms of illness, great variations can exist in one's level of health and vitality. In other words, your vast potential for experiencing physical, mental and emotional well-being cannot be adequately described simply as an absence of illness. The term "wellness" refers to this great positive potential.

The graph shown below can help to illustrate the idea of wellness. In it, the mid-point—represented by zero—symbolizes the borderline between illness and the absence of illness. Above this seemingly neutral point rises a broad range of positive potential for enhanced well-being; below it looms the gruesome spectre of creeping illness and gradual loss of ability.

From top to bottom, the scale ranges from what you might consider to be your ideal state of health, fitness and well-being, at +10, to a minimum state of wellness at -10.

Mark the point on the scale to the right which you feel best represents your overall condition today—that is, your present state of wellness and vitality.

Next, think back in time to a period about five years ago. Get an image of your condition at that time. Now mark the point on the scale to the left which you feel best represents your overall condition as of five years ago.

Connect these two points with an arrow directed from your past to your present condition. This arrow indicates the direction of your recent health history as you have experienced it.

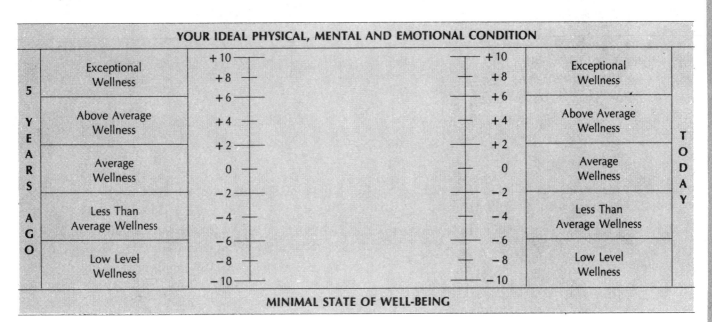

The Lifestyle Inventory will assist you to project a greater measure of wellness into your future.

MEASURE YOUR PRESENT CONDITION

Your Body Composition

You may use these guidelines to determine your ideal weight:

Adult male: Allow 106 pounds for the first five feet of height, and add 6 pounds for each additional inch.

Adult female: Allow 100 pounds for the first five feet of height, and add 5 pounds for each additional inch.

Adjustment for Frame Size: Subtract 10% from these results if you have a light frame; add 10% for a heavy frame.

YOUR PRESENT WEIGHT   _____

DIVIDED BY YOUR IDEAL WEIGHT   ÷ _____

EQUALS   = _____

MINUS   − 1.00

EQUALS PERCENT OVERWEIGHT   = _____

Enter the score from the table that matches your percent overweight.   _____
YOUR SCORE
from the table

Note: Many people, if they are in good physical condition at the time, achieve a desirable weight between the ages of 18 and 23.

Percent Overweight	Your Score	Your Weight Tends To Support
0	50	Exceptional Wellness
1 to 2	47	Exceptional Wellness
3 to 4	44	
5 to 6	41	Above Average Wellness
7 to 9	38	
10 to 13	35	Average Wellness
14 to 19	32	
20 to 26	29	Less Than Average Wellness
27 to 33	26	
34 to 50	23	Low Level Wellness
over 75	20	

Your Resting Heart Rate

How fast your heart beats when you are at rest indicates how hard your heart has to work simply to maintain your basic body functions. This, in turn, is a useful indicator of the fitness of your heart, lungs, blood and blood vessels.

Your resting heart rate may be measured after you have been sitting or lying in a relaxed state for five minutes or so. To determine your heart rate, place the second and third fingers along the thumb side of the opposite wrist, and count the pulsations for one minute.

YOUR RESTING HEART RATE _____

Enter the score from the table that matches your resting heart rate.   _____
YOUR SCORE
from the table

Resting Heart Rate	Your Score	Your Rate Tends To Support
under 50	50	Exceptional Wellness
50 to 54	47	Exceptional Wellness
55 to 59	44	
60 to 64	41	Above Average Wellness
65 to 68	38	
69 to 72	35	Average Wellness
73 to 76	32	
77 to 80	29	Less Than Average Wellness
81 to 84	26	
85 to 88	23	Low Level Wellness
over 88	20	

Your Smoking History

Circle the score beside the one statement that best describes your experience with smoking.

   0   I have never smoked, or I quit smoking more than 15 years ago.

− 1   I quit smoking 10 to 15 years ago.

− 2   I quit smoking 5 to 10 years ago.

− 3   I quit smoking less than 5 years ago.

− 20   I presently smoke 1 to 7 cigarettes per day.

− 23   I presently smoke 8 to 14 cigarettes per day or I smoke cigars or a pipe.

− 26   I presently smoke 15 to 25 cigarettes per day.

− 30   I presently smoke more than 25 cigarettes per day.

Circle the score beside *each* statement that is true for you.

− 2   I have lived with a person who smokes during 2 or more of the past 4 years.

− 2   I have worked in a smoky area during 2 or more of the past 4 years.

− 1   I have lived in a high smog area during 2 or more of the past 4 years.

Add up your smoking history scores and enter the total here.   − _____
YOUR   SCORE

SUMMARIZE YOUR PRESENT CONDITION

**Summarize your Present Condition by adding up
the three scores you've developed so far.**

Your BODY COMPOSITION SCORE   +_____

PLUS: Your RESTING HEART RATE SCORE   +_____

EQUALS: Subtotal   =_____

MINUS: Your SMOKING HISTORY SCORE   −_____

YOUR PRESENT CONDITION SCORE   =_____

Mark Your Score Here	Your Patterns Tend To Support
	Exceptional Wellness
86	
	Above Average Wellness
72	
	Average Wellness
58	
	Less Than Average Wellness
44	
	Low Level Wellness

The sections to follow explore a number of ways in which your Present Condition is being shaped by your lifestyle.

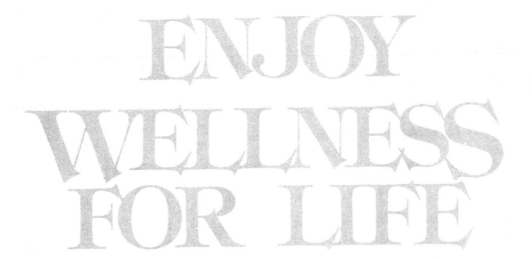

ENJOY WELLNESS FOR LIFE

MEASURE YOUR LIFESTYLE

For each of the following questions, mark one of the squares beside the single answer that is most correct for you at this time. (Two columns of squares are provided so that you can note your responses on two separate occasions. On each such occasion, be sure to mark all of your answers in the same column.)

Your Stress Management Patterns

CLARITY AND PERSONAL ORGANIZATION

In my present life situation:

☐ ☐ **3** I feel confined and unable to express myself as I would like.

☐ ☐ **6** I feel somewhat limited.

☐ ☐ **9** I am able to be the person I choose to be, and to do the things I enjoy most.

In areas where I have expectations:

☐ ☐ **3** in one or more key matters, I frequently fear undesired outcomes.

☐ ☐ **6** my expectations are sometimes clouded with doubt regarding my ability to be, do or have as I would like.

☐ ☐ **9** In general, I clearly see myself thinking, feeling and behaving just as I most truly choose to be.

When I feel that I have been slighted, offended or somehow harmed by the actions of another:

☐ ☐ **3** I tend to remain angry, resentful and bitter, hoping that somehow the score can be evened.

☐ ☐ **6** I generally excuse others for their errors and omissions, chalking it up to their ignorance or incompetence.

☐ ☐ **9** I consistently choose to unconditionally forgive any harmful words or actions by others, thus freeing myself for fully effective action, unburdened by blameful thoughts or destructive emotions.

When working on tasks which demand concentration:

☐ ☐ **3** I am frequently distracted by other matters.

☐ ☐ **6** I have some difficulty staying focused on what I'm doing.

☐ ☐ **9** I can usually stay focused on what I'm doing without undue distraction.

Regarding my sense of responsibility:

☐ ☐ **3** I generally feel responsible for everything that is going on.

☐ ☐ **6** I often feel responsible for situations and events that are beyond my control.

☐ ☐ **9** I feel responsible for assuring that my thoughts, feelings and behavior represent me at my very best, and that my conduct is fully harmonized with my values, intuitions and most noble intentions.

ATTITUDE CONTROL

Regarding personal achievement, I am:

☐ ☐ **3** constantly driven to work harder in order to measure up to my own high standards.

☐ ☐ **6** somewhat pressured to work harder in order to prove myself.

☐ ☐ **9** relaxed, confident that I am responding appropriately to my circumstances.

When I am working against a tight schedule:

☐ ☐ **3** I am often nervous, and frequently become impatient with delays.

☐ ☐ **6** I am sometimes nervous, and occasionally become impatient with delays.

☐ ☐ **9** I generally remain calm, responding to delays with patience and renewed determination.

Regarding my need for information:

☐ ☐ **3** I become very uncomfortable when I don't know exactly what is going on.

☐ ☐ **6** I feel somewhat uncomfortable with uncertainty and try hard to eliminate the unknowns.

☐ ☐ **9** I can live with uncertainty, even enjoying the adventure of facing the unknown.

When the assistance of others could aid me in getting my needs met:

☐ ☐ 3   I often expect them to be unresponsive to me, and may not even bother to request their help.

☐ ☐ 6   I often expect others to be at least somewhat reluctant to assist me, and plan to get what I want through pleading, trickery, intimidation or force.

☐ ☐ 9   I generally expect others to be supportive and cooperative once I have brought my needs to their attention.

My satisfaction and sense of accomplishment are derived from:

☐ ☐ 3   mainly the rewards and recognition I receive from others.

☐ ☐ 6   sometimes my own appreciation; more often the recognition I receive from others.

☐ ☐ 9   mainly the personal knowledge that I have performed to be best of my ability.

My interests are:

☐ ☐ 3   mostly confined to matters which are related to my work.

☐ ☐ 6   somewhat varied.

☐ ☐ 9   numerous and varied, including areas that are quite unrelated to my work.

With regard to expressing my feelings:

☐ ☐ 3   I keep my true feelings to myself in most situations.

☐ ☐ 6   I find it somewhat difficult to express my real feelings.

☐ ☐ 9   I find it easy to express my feelings in most situations.

In dealing with my deepest personal concerns.

☐ ☐ 3   I feel unable to discuss my most difficult problems with anyone.

☐ ☐ 6   sometimes I feel I have no one to talk with about what's really bothering me.

☐ ☐ 9   I have trusted persons with whom I can usually discuss whatever is on my mind.

When others are speaking to me:

☐ ☐ 3   I'm often thinking of what I'm going to say next, and frequently interrupt the speaker.

☐ ☐ 6   I listen intermittently, sometimes interrupting the speaker with my own thoughts.

☐ ☐ 9   I usually listen attentively, rarely interrupting the speaker.

The quality of my sleep is:

☐ ☐ 3   often disturbed by anxious thoughts or distressing dreams.

☐ ☐ 6   sometimes sound; other times disturbed.

☐ ☐ 9   sound, peaceful and refreshing; undisturbed by the concerns of the day.

CONSCIOUS RELAXATION

I reduce the effect of stress in my life by engaging in some method of conscious relaxation:

☐ ☐ 25   infrequently – once a week or less.

☐ ☐ 50   occasionally – every few days.

☐ ☐ 75   almost every day.

Add up your stress management scores for your current set of responses and enter the total here.

YOUR STRESS MANAGEMENT SCORE _____ _____

Mark Your Score Here		Your Patterns Tend To Support:
		Exceptional Wellness
168		Above Average Wellness
140		Average Wellness
112		Less Than Average Wellness
84		Low Level Wellness

Your Physical Activity Patterns

FULL-BODY STRETCHES

I perform full-body stretches to maintain my flexibility and range of motion:

☐ ☐ **20** once a week or less.

☐ ☐ **40** every few days.

☐ ☐ **60** almost every day.

CARDIO-RESPIRATORY ACTIVITY

An "aerobic workout" consists of five essential parts:

first, a brief pre-exercise stretch;
second, a short warm-up period;
third, at least 12 minutes of continuous activity which is sufficiently vigorous to maintain your heart rate at 80 percent of its maximum for your age;
fourth, a short cool-down period; and
fifth, a brief post-exercise stretch.

I provide my body with a complete, five-part aerobic workout:

☐ ☐ **40** once a week or less.

☐ ☐ **80** two or three times a week.

☐ ☐ **120** more than three times a week.

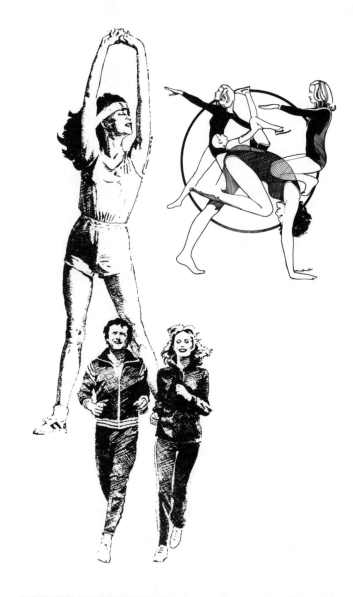

BODY-TONING

I engage in activities which help me to maintain the tone and strength of my major muscles and bones:

☐ ☐ **10** once a week or less.

☐ ☐ **20** one or two times a week.

☐ ☐ **30** three or more times each week.

Add up your physical activity scores for your current set of responses and enter the total here:

YOUR PHYSICAL ACTIVITY SCORE _____ _____

Mark Your Score Here		Your Patterns Tend To Support:
		Exceptional Wellness
170		Above Average Wellness
140		Average Wellness
110		Less Than Average Wellness
80		Low Level Wellness

Your Nutritional Patterns

EATING INDEPENDENCE

I feel that the quantity of food I eat *at meals* is:

☐ ☐ **10** frequent excessive — I usually don't stop eating until I feel full.

☐ ☐ **20** occasionally excessive.

☐ ☐ **30** rarely excessive — I usually finish eating before feeling full.

I feel that the eating and drinking I do — *aside from meals* — is:

☐ ☐ **10** frequent; substantial; high fat or sugar.

☐ ☐ **20** occasional; moderate.

☐ ☐ **30** infrequent; insubstantial; unrefined carbohydrates.

UNREFINED CARBOHYDRATES INTAKE
(vegetables, fruit, whole grains)

I eat fresh fruit:

☐ ☐ **5** infrequently — many days none at all.

☐ ☐ **10** occasionally — many days I get some.

☐ ☐ **15** once or twice almost every day.

I eat leafy green vegetables:

☐ ☐ **10** infrequently — many days none at all.

☐ ☐ **20** occasionally — many days I get some.

☐ ☐ **30** once or twice almost every day.

I eat other vegetables such as beans, potatoes, peas, lentils, squash and yams.

☐ ☐ **5** infrequently — many days none at all.

☐ ☐ **10** occasionally — many days I get some.

☐ ☐ **15** almost every day.

The wheat and other grains I eat are mostly:

☐ ☐ **5** highly processed, bleached white.

☐ ☐ **10** medium processed, enriched whole wheat.

☐ ☐ **15** coarse ground, whole grain.

FAT INTAKE

The meats that I eat are mostly:

☐ ☐ **10** high fat — pork, prime beef, hamburger, organ meats, duck, lamb, etc.

☐ ☐ **20** medium fat — lean beef, veal, chicken and turkey with skin.

☐ ☐ **30** lean — fish, chicken and turkey without skin, or no meat at all.

The dairy products that I consume are mostly:

☐ ☐ **5** high fat — whole milk, cream, cheddar and other full-fat cheeses.

☐ ☐ **10** low fat.

☐ ☐ **15** skim milk, low fat cheeses, or no dairy products at all.

I eat deep-fried foods, including most fast foods:

☐ ☐ **5** often — three or more times a week.

☐ ☐ **10** occasionally — about twice a week.

☐ ☐ **15** seldom — once a week or less.

Regarding fats such as butter, margarine, mayonnaise, salad dressings and oils:

☐ ☐ **5** I don't control my intake.

☐ ☐ **10** I eat 3 or 4 teaspoons per day.

☐ ☐ **15** I eat 2 teaspoons or less per day.

Add up your nutritional scores for your current set of responses and enter the total here:

YOUR NUTRITIONAL SCORE _____ _____

Mark Your Score Here		Your Patterns Tend To Support:
		Exceptional Wellness
170		Above Average Wellness
140		Average Wellness
110		Less Than Average Wellness
80		Low Level Wellness

Chemical Independence

CAFFEINE

My average daily consumption of caffeine drinks, including coffee, non-herbal tea, cocoa, cola and chocolate is:

☐ ☐   **0**   one cup or less.

☐ ☐ **− 5**   two or three cups.

☐ ☐ **− 10**   four or more cups.

ALCOHOL

The amount of alcohol I consume averages *(standard serving = 12 oz beer; 4 oz wine; 1-1/4 oz whiskey)***:**

☐ ☐   **0**   one standard serving per day or less of any alcoholic beverage.

☐ ☐ **− 10**   two standard servings per day.

☐ ☐ **− 40**   three or more standard servings per day.

DRUG INDEPENDENCE

I use other mood altering substances:

☐ ☐   **0**   seldom or never.

☐ ☐ **− 10**   occasionally − less than once a week.

☐ ☐ **− 20**   frequently − once a week or more.

With regard to both prescription and over-the-counter medications:

☐ ☐   **0**   I take as little as possible, and then only as directed.

☐ ☐ **− 10**   I take quite a bit, sometimes simply for "extra insurance."

☐ ☐ **− 20**   I take a lot, whether or not it is clearly necessary at the time; or, I take them in unapproved combinations.

TOBACCO

With regard to tobacco:

☐ ☐   **0**   I am a non-smoker.

☐ ☐ **− 50**   I use tobacco.

Add up your chemical independence scores for your current set of responses and enter the total here.

YOUR CHEMICAL INDEPENDENCE SCORE _____ _____

Mark Your Score Here		Your Patterns Tend To Support:
0		Exceptional Wellness
0		Above Average Wellness
−18		Average Wellness
−25		Less Than Average Wellness
		Low Level Wellness

SUMMARIZE YOUR LIFESTYLE

Summarize your Lifestyle Inventory by adding up your total scores from the preceding lifestyle measurements.

	Your STRESS MANAGEMENT SCORE (from page 9)	+_____	+_____
PLUS:	Your PHYSICAL ACTIVITY SCORE (from page 10)	+_____	+_____
PLUS:	Your NUTRITIONAL SCORE (from page 11)	+_____	+_____
EQUALS:	Subtotal	=_____	=_____
MINUS:	Your CHEMICAL INDEPENDENCE SCORE (from page 12)	−_____	−_____
EQUALS:	**YOUR LIFESTYLE SCORE**	=_____	=_____

Then enter your **PRESENT CONDITION SCORE** (page 7) _____

Your Present Condition Score Supports	Your Present Condition Score		Your Lifestyle Score	Your Lifestyle Score Supports
Exceptional Wellness	93		547	Exceptional Wellness
	86		503	
Above Average Wellness	79		464	Above Average Wellness
	72		419	
Average Wellness	65		366	Average Wellness
	58		336	
Less Than Average Wellness	51		274	Less Than Average Wellness
	44		225	
Low Level Wellness	37		67	Low Level Wellness

Place a mark representing your PRESENT CONDITION SCORE (from page 7) on the scale to the left.

Place a second mark, representing your LIFESTYLE SCORE (from page 12) on the scale to the right.

Connect these two points with an arrow pointing from your PRESENT CONDITION mark to your LIFESTYLE mark.

This arrow gives a general indication of the influence your present lifestyle might be expected to exert on your level of wellness with the passage of time.

Consult with your physician to develop an even more comprehensive picture of your present condition, and to obtain his or her assistance in establishing a safe and effective strategy for improving your overall state of health.

Now that you've had a look at your living patterns and how they relate to your wellness, where do you go from here?

The remainder of this workbook is designed to help you answer this question for yourself. It provides information related to each of the lifestyle factors contained in the inventory, and offers an opportunity for you to design an enjoyable, wellness-oriented personal lifestyle for yourself.

Maintaining wellness for life begins with stress management because the powerful stress response influences virtually every aspect of your experience, including:

- your awareness of who you are and of your true intent with respect to all the situations you encounter;
- where you place your attention;
- how you feel, what you see and hear, and, consequently, what you perceive;
- your interpretation and judgment of events;
- the nature of your recollections;
- the future which you envision and expect;
- your attitude toward yourself and the world in which you live;
- your ultimate self-expression in gesture, word and deed.

With positive stress management you can harness these fundamental forces and put them to constructive work in your life.

The early effects of chronic unrelieved stress may include headaches, stomach upsets, sleeplessness, hypertension, lower back pain, psychosomatic illnesses, anxiety, irritability, mental disorientation, smoking, alcohol and drug abuse.

Longer term effects may include heart disease, stroke, cancer, ulcers, narrowing and hardening of the arteries, obesity and alcoholism. The extent of the problem is reflected in the fact that valium, which temporarily masks some of the symptoms of acute distress, is one of the most prescribed drugs in the world today.

Stress management amounts to taking control of yourself. Not in an impatient, critical and punitive sense, but in a caring, compassionate, yet firmly determined sense.

Stress management means taking good care of yourself, and appreciating yourself for who you are. Not because you've earned it, but because you are, by your nature, deserving of respect and appreciation. From this central point of strength, you can extend your attitude of peace, acceptance, appreciation, confidence and determination, first to others, and then to the entire world of your personal experience.

What Is Stress?

Your body responds, sometimes dramatically, to each of your emotions. Its natural response to fear is to mobilize for efficient defensive action with the so-called *"fight-or-flight" response.* At the extreme, this is what happens:

- once your brain is activated, it calls for release of chemicals into the blood-stream which signal an emergency to the rest of your body;
- your chest expands to draw more oxygen into your lungs;
- your heart and blood vessels dilate, and your blood pressure rises to accelerate the flow of vital fluids throughout your body;
- your liver releases glucose into the bloodstream to fuel your muscles;
- your muscles contract in preparation for immediate movement;
- your skin surface blood vessels contract, causing your skin to pale;
- your blood is enriched with coagulants to quickly stop the bleeding if your skin is punctured;
- your pupils dilate and your eyelids open to maximize visual input;
- perspiration increases, goose bumps form and your hair stands on end to improve body cooling;
- your bladder and intestines may empty themselves of unnecessary matter.

Many seemingly superhuman feats are accomplished when the vast resources of the body are mobilized in this extraordinary way. In one well publicized example, a woman was actually able to lift an automobile from her injured child.

Marvelous as it is, this response can do great damage to your body when it is not given adequate release. Yet hard running and physical defense are seldom called for in dealing with the typical challenges of modern living, such as job pressures, financial uncertainties, family and social obligations, and more generalized cultural concerns like environmental deterioration and the nuclear threat. Chronic, low grade stimulation of your powerful fight-or-flight response has detrimental effects on your body's regulatory, nervous, circulatory and immunological systems.

Fortunately stress is not an inherent quality of your external circumstances. It is a response to your circumstances which takes place inside of you, and is therefore subject to your personal control. This is evident from the great differences observable among individual responses to the same set of circumstances.

You can break the hold of chronic stress with these three strategies:

1. Regularly practice conscious relaxation.

2. Continuously maintain your clarity and personal organization.

3. Exercise positive attitude control.

Conscious Relaxation

The physiological responses associated with stress and anxiety are incompatible with deep muscle relaxation. This means that by fully relaxing your entire body, and along with it your mind and emotions, you can break the hold of chronic stress, diminishing its influence upon your body and your life. Interestingly, conscious relaxation has stress reducing effects that cannot be provided by simply sitting quietly or even by sleeping. Your body waits to be told that it's safe to relax; otherwise, it may faithfully hold itself in a state of perpetual readiness, regardless of what you may be doing.

The regular practice of conscious relaxation also develops the essential skills which underlie both powerful personal goal-setting, and reliable attitude control. To do either with full effectiveness requires cultivation of your ability to interrupt and divert the continual flow of imagery, or self-talk, which otherwise passes automatically across the field of your consciousness. Taking positive control of your life implies a growing facility for channeling your thoughts, and thereby your emotions and actions, in the directions that you choose for yourself when you are at your very best.

Conscious relaxation is a simple process in which first your body, and then your mind and emotions, are gradually brought to a point of silence—a tranquil state which is then purposefully maintained for a short period of time. At the end of this quiet period, you are ideally situated for your goal clarification activity, free of any conflicting thoughts, feelings or sensations. As you become more adept in the practice of quieting your mind, your capacity for making instantaneous adjustments in your attitude will also grow.

This conscious relaxation procedure is adapted from extensive research conducted by Herbert Benson, M.D., and reported in his best-selling book "The Relaxation Response." It is an effective method of releasing yourself from the grip of chronic tension.

1. Select a place where you will not be disturbed. Sit quietly in a comfortable position with your eyes closed.

2. Deeply relax all your muscles by placing your attention upon them one at a time, beginning with the muscles of your feet and working all the way up to the muscles of your face. Allow your body to remain relaxed.

3. Breathe through your nose. Become aware of your breathing, and as you breathe out, say a single word or phrase silently to yourself. This phrase can be neutral in meaning, such as the word "one," or it can be any other expression which has a calming and empowering effect upon you. Continue observing your breathing, while repeating your chosen word or phrase to yourself with each exhalation. Do this for at least five minutes at the outset, gradually lengthening your period of conscious relaxation to as long as twenty minutes. You may open your eyes to check the time, but do not use an alarm. After you finish, sit quietly for awhile, at first with your eyes closed, then with them open.

Don't worry about whether you are successful in achieving a "deep level of relaxation." Just maintain a receptive attitude and permit relaxation to occur at its own pace. Expect other thoughts, and allow them to pass undisturbed when they occur. Simply breathe them out with a quiet "one." With practice, full relaxation will come to you without effort.

A convenient way of reducing stress that can be practiced at any time and in any place is to take several deep breaths. Concentrate on inhaling and exhaling slowly, with your mouth closed. Slowly breathe in until you can't take in any more air, then slowly exhale until you've squeezed every last bit of air from your lungs.

Stress inclines you to breathe in short, shallow breaths, whereas deep breathing provides you with maximum oxygen and virtually forces you to relax.

When you fully relax yourself once or twice each day, you open the door to taking positive control over every other aspect of your life. If you are not already accustomed to engaging in some form of conscious relaxation, begin now by setting a specific time for it each day, allowing at least 10 minutes per session at the outset. Pick a convenient time, considering your current schedule, and then enter these periods onto your Planning Calendar (page 4).

Goal Clarity and Personal Organization

Successful stress management involves setting your own directions by establishing worthwhile goals for yourself.

Your goals need to be **realistic** in the sense that they effectively address the actual circumstances of your life. At the same time, they need to be **idealistic** in the sense that they truly encompass your highest aspirations, and properly reflect your noblest intent. Make it a point to insist that each of your goals incorporates this harmonious blend of practical realism and genuinely rewarding idealism. Though at times this may require a bit of creative energy, you'll soon discover that it's never necessary to set your sights on anything less than what you really want most.

Clarity and personal organization are the product of a continuous process, involving the sorting out of confusions, the reduction of uncertainty and doubt, and the constructive rechanneling of reactive emotions such as fear, anger, hatred, envy or guilt.

The more simply and concretely you can state your goals, the better. To develop a clear image of your goals for yourself, use as many of your faculties as possible. For example, in addition to **seeing** the realization of your goals, you gain even greater clarity and certainty by **feeling** what it's like for them to be fulfilled, and by **accepting** them as already accomplished within the realm of your creative imagination.

In carrying out these goal clarification exercises, visualize everything in the present, and state your goals to yourself in the present, rather than in the future. In this way you are able to give yourself a more complete experience of what it's like to have already accomplished the task that you have set for yourself. This enables you to further specify your goal, and prepares you for the experience of realizing it.

Begin your goal clarification exercises by relaxing yourself in a comfortable position where you will not be disturbed. A good time may be immediately following your period of conscious relaxation.

Close your eyes and then see, feel and accept yourself as already **being** the person you choose to be. Visualize yourself in as much detail as possible, relating honorably and effectively to the realities of your current life situation. Use your imagination and enjoy yourself.

Next see and feel yourself **doing** what you choose to do, again in as much detail as possible. Then see and feel what it's like to **enjoy having** the things that come with being and doing as you have chosen.

This exercise creates a well-rounded picture of your goal in very specific, concrete and personal terms. It specifies your inner state of being—your identity, as well as your behavior, and your outer environment—what you have.

In accomplishing these exercises, don't allow any negative self-talk to enter in. At this point you are not attempting to figure out **how** to achieve your goal. You are simply identifying what the goal is. This is the time to reveal and eliminate any negative, self-defeating assumptions that you may have been laboring under.

Action planning

After your goals have been clearly established, you are ready to prepare any necessary action plans, along with timetables for the completion of key steps. Make sure that all your planning is directed toward the practical realization of the goals you have set for yourself. Specify the actual steps that you intend to take in achieving your goals. To be realistic, the steps must logically lead from wherever you are right now to the ultimate realization of your goals.

In order for your goals to be practically useful to you in the present, they must be stated in concrete terms that are responsive to your immediate circumstances, and respectful of your true potential as an individual.

Maintain a worthy set of goals. Staying on track in all the important areas of life is aided by having a clear image of what you would like. Here are a few areas that you may wish to attend to from time to time, making certain that your goals are clear:

- Relationships with family and friends.
- Relationships with co-workers.
- Occupational activities and aspirations.
- Financial activities and goals.
- Recreational activities and interests.
- Environmental quality in your home, at work, and in your community.

The more clearly you are able to specify your true preferences with respect to the key circumstances of your life, the more likely you are to experience their ultimate fulfillment.

It's only common sense, yet all too easily forgotten when your attention is captivated by your circumstances, as can so easily happen when you are "under stress."

When you truly experience yourself as already being the person you choose to be, your behavior tends to become consistent with this new self-image.

In this way you're not fighting yourself for a change in behavior. Instead, the desired behavior flows naturally from your newly adopted self-concept.

Clarity and personal organization are the necessary underpinnings for effective functioning on a moment-by-moment basis in the course of your daily affairs. Check yourself regularly to assure that you are enjoying a clear sense of who you are and where you're headed with respect to all the important areas of your life. There's no need to live with nagging dissatisfactions and chronic feelings of helplessness when you can far more easily turn your experience around with a bit of determination and creative problem solving.

Attitude Control

With your self-image and direction clearly established, the next step is to make sure that you're staying on track in the course of your daily affairs. Having already privately experienced your preferences with respect to all the key situations in your life, you're well prepared to enjoy the rewarding experience of living them out.

Attitude control is your moment by moment choice of orientation with respect to the ever-shifting circumstances of life. At each point in time, you may either act in accordance with your conscious choice, or fall back upon previously developed habit patterns. Ordinarily the choice is easy, and your prior visualizations place you in the perfect position to smoothly realize your preferences.

However, when a perceived threat arises, it may trigger the physiologically compelling "fight-or-flight" response, which in turn tends to throw your entire system into a more or less automatic reaction. Under these conditions, your spontaneous thought and behavior will tend to reflect the patterns which you have habitually associated with the feelings prevailing at that time.

It is at precisely these moments that your awareness of who you are can be called to your aid. Recognize yourself as the author of your life, take a deep breath, relax your body, quiet your mind, still your emotions, and insert your preferred self-image directly into the flow of experience. In this manner you will be able to restore your full capacity for noble and effective action.

Chronic stress is associated with specific attitudes and behaviors. These include: impatience, inability to relax without feeling anxious or guilty, excessive competitiveness, aggressiveness (as opposed to assertiveness), inability to listen attentively without thinking of other things, a reliance upon external rewards and recognition for the maintenance of self-esteem, an immoderate need for information and control, a pervasive sense of personal responsibility, and a highly judgmental attitude.

On the positive side, there's a set of corresponding attitudes and behaviors which are not only highly effective, but also conducive to lasting good health. For example, the much admired ability to remain calm, self-possessed and efficient in a tight situation. Or the ability to listen attentively and empathetically to others when they are speaking. There's also being supportive of others and rejoicing in their successes, rather than indulging in jealous competition. Or being able to humbly acknowledge your true feelings and to discuss those matters that are of greatest importance to you. Others include thoroughly enjoying the experience of living and being human, quite apart from the gratifications of external rewards and recognition; and appreciating yourself and others for having performed at your personal peak, aside from any comparative results which may come from your actions.

Your goal clarification activities are ideally suited for installing these and other positive attributes as characteristic traits of your personality. In addition, you can exercise attitude control to handle those cases in which your observed response

*A word of caution...*don't allow planning considerations to discourage you from continuing to pursue your ultimate goals. To do so would be equivalent to a young person deciding not to become a physician because he or she doesn't have a car to get to school with. The purpose of goal setting is to determine where you are going, whereas the purpose of planning is to set a suitable course for getting there.

Self Efficacy

In order for your goals to be truly realistic and your plans practically achievable, you must believe that you can, in fact, accomplish them. Perhaps the single most influential factor in determining the success of any particular plan is your perception of yourself as actually being capable of executing it. The important thing to remember is that this "self-efficacy" is bestowed by you upon yourself. While it is indeed encouraging when other people believe in your ability, success in life is likely to frequently require that you generate your own sense of competence in areas that are important to you.

Use your conscious relaxation skills and goal clarification exercises to build your sense of competence whenever you notice that you doubt your ability to achieve what you really feel is best for you and for those you serve.

Stress tends to place you in a reactive relationship to your circumstances, while effective stress management puts you in control of yourself with respect to your circumstances.

Practice a virtue a day.

Benjamin Franklin made it a point to practice one particular virtue each day. Effective attitude control can be aided by focusing on a variety of desirable attributes, one at a time. Here are a few areas which you may want to attend to. Add more as you feel the need.

- Openness, friendliness, attentiveness.
- Honesty, forthrightness, expressiveness.
- Playfulness, spontaneity, enjoyment of life.
- Humor, sense of perspective, appreciation of the lighter side of things.
- Forgiveness.
- Appreciation of self and others.
- Confidence in self and others.
- Positive recollections of past events.
- Patience, tolerance of delays, imperfections and disappointments.
- Determination and persistence in the pursuit of your worthwhile goals.
- Assistance to others, supportiveness, cooperation.
- Concentration on whatever task is at hand.
- Caring for others, exercising compassionate understanding of self and others.

Obstacles to successful attitude control are habitual patterns of negative self-talk. Your attitudes are shaped by what you say to yourself in your ongoing mental conversation. The private "movies" you play for yourself while driving home from work or while taking a shower fortify your position within the world of your experience. Begin watching this flow of imagery from a positive, stress management point of view, inserting the kinds of suggestions you'd like to see yourself living out. Learn to expect the best—from yourself, from others, and from the world in general. Anxiety gives way to enthusiasm with increasing mastery of life.

to a situation is inconsistent with your preferences. For example, you may choose to be a patient, compassionate person, yet observe yourself becoming impatient and highly critical.

Fortunately, at this point you have already taken the first, most crucial step in exercising control over your attitude—that is, you have become aware of what you are doing. Your natural response upon making such an observation might be to turn your impatience and criticism back in upon yourself, thereby even further complicating matters. Instead of directly opposing what you are doing, provide yourself with a suitable alternative to the course you are on.

Establish an appropriate perspective. What seems important at the moment very often pales to insignificance when viewed within a broader context. You might briefly consider how important this event is likely to appear to you after a year or two has passed. This will help establish the proper relationship between the momentary events at hand and the larger scale of your life.

Pay attention to what is going on, without passing judgment on any aspect of what is taking place. Notice what is happening as an interested observer, without drawing conclusions, and without attempting to justify, explain or criticize.

From this position of detached observation, you are far more likely to become aware of all the options available to you in relating to the situation at hand, including your preferred ways of thinking, feeling and behaving. And here is where your preparatory goal clarification work can really pay off. In many cases, a tasteful touch of good humor may be all that's needed to immediately transform the entire situation from tense to relaxed. The key point is that you are acting in accordance with your conscious choice, rather than remaining bound within an unpleasant chain of unrewarding reactions.

In summary, by consciously relaxing yourself on a regular basis, by remaining aware of who you are and where you are going, and by keeping yourself on track, you can constructively manage your response to the normal stresses of life.

Keep an eye on your progress

The Living Well Daily Performance Log, which appears on page 60, provides you with a means of systematically reviewing your progress in all the key areas of wellness.

For each of the three Stress Management areas, simply fill in the appropriate circles for the day in question. At the end of the week, you'll be able to summarize your activities, so that you can then transfer the weekly information to your Long-Term Progress Record (page 67).

DAILY PERFORMANCE RECORD — WEEK 1

		OBJECTIVE		S	M	T	W	T	F	S	#	X	=	TOTAL
STRESS MANAGEMENT	A	Clarity and Personal Organization	clear & organized	○	○	○	○	○	○	○		45		
			a bit disorganized	○	○	○	○	○	○	○		30		
			poorly organized	○	○	○	○	○	○	○		15		
	B	Attitude Control	positive attitude	○	○	○	○	○	○	○		90		
			mostly positive	○	○	○	○	○	○	○		60		
			negative attitude	○	○	○	○	○	○	○		30		
	C	Conscious Relaxation	at least 5 minutes	○	○	○	○	○	○	○		75		
			less than 5 minutes	○	○	○	○	○	○	○		25		

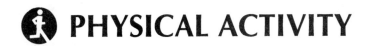

Your body—the hundred trillion celled organism supporting your personal awareness—has amazing potential for movement and manipulation of its environment. It's up to you to actualize this potential, for without regular use, your body tends to become stiff, weak, and sluggish.

While such losses are often viewed as the inevitable consequences of aging, proper physical activity can help to reduce the decline of your strength, flexibility and endurance to less than 15 percent between the ages of 20 and 60. And if you were out of shape at 20, you may actually be stronger at 60.

Your body directly reflects the demands which you place upon it. Each day billions of your body cells die and billions more are produced according to the demands of your current activity patterns and the quality of your nutritional intake.

A fully effective exercise program activates three distinct physical potentials: your muscle and joint flexibility, your cardio-respiratory capacity, and the strength and balance of your muscles and bones.

Flexibility

The first component of a well-rounded program of physical activity is full-body stretching. Everyone is familiar with the richly satisfying feeling of a good stretch after a prolonged period of physical inactivity. **You can easily maintain your flexibility and range of motion with a simple routine of regular, systematic stretching.** At least once each day, give your body a complete stretch.

The key to successful physical development in all areas is progression. In the case of stretching, this means extending and flexing your muscles and joints only to the limits of your personal comfort—never beyond. Perform your stretches in a slow, gentle manner. Breathe deeply while stretching, letting go of a little more tension with each exhalation. You'll be amazed at how your flexibility increases with regular, patient, easy stretching. Specific stretching exercises to help you cover all your major joints and muscles are provided on pages 26, 27 and 28.

In addition to maintaining the flexibility and range of motion of your major muscles and joints, stretching is a necessary preliminary to safely performing both aerobic and body toning activities. So if you're planning to begin with just one of the three types of recommended activity, then daily full-body stretching is a natural way to get started.

Choose a convenient time for your daily stretch—perhaps upon arising in the morning, or in the quiet of the evening, or just prior to any aerobic or body toning workouts you have planned. Performing the 17 recommended daily stretches for 15 to 30 seconds each takes just ten minutes a day. Enter these periods into your Planning Calendar on page 4.

Cardio-Respiratory Capacity

The second component of an effective exercise program maintains and expands your cardio-respiratory capacity.

Each of your cells needs a constant supply of fuel and oxygen to give you the energy and stamina you need to get the most out of life. Your body is renewed and energized by the efficient operation of the system that feeds your cells—the cardio-respiratory system composed of your lungs, heart, blood and blood vessels. The more efficiently oxygen is absorbed into your bloodstream and

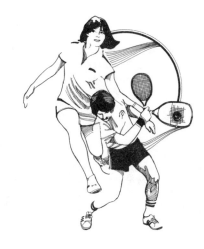

One of the keys to maintaining an effective pattern of physical activity is to find one or more activities that you truly enjoy, and then sticking with them, perfecting your skills and developing your interest.

Some potential benefits of a well-designed exercise program are...

Greater: strength
    endurance
    flexibility
    vitality
Reduced: muscle tension
    anxiety
    depression
    boredom
    mental fatigue
Improved: muscle tone
    bone density
    metabolism
    weight control
Lower risk of: heart and arterial disease
    low back pain
    sleep disorders

In addition, regular exercise may increase your productivity and heighten your enjoyment of work. It may also provide you with an enhanced sense of well-being and self-confidence.

Indeed, proper physical activity can add a lot to the quality of your life, and inactivity can take a heavy toll.

Your lungs are a honeycomb of passages opening to a thousand square feet of surface area—20 times more than your outer skin. This gives your blood exposure to the atmosphere, so it can exhaust waste carbon dioxide and absorb fresh oxygen.

Your heart pumps more than 5 quarts of blood every minute; 2,000 gallons a day in 10,000 pulsations. The unfit system requires the heart to work 20-30 percent harder just to meet minimal demands. In a year that's 10 million extra beats by an engine that has to last a lifetime.

Your blood vessels are a 60,000 mile labyrinth of tubing distributed throughout your body. When elastic and unobstructed, they can channel blood at speeds up to 50 miles per hour.

Your bloodstream is refreshed with a billion new red blood cells every day. The continued health of your heart and blood vessels depends upon maintaining a balance among certain blood components. For example, too much of the wrong kind of fat clogs the pores in the artery walls, eventually building up layers of plaque which limit the flow of vital fluids.

transported throughout your body, the more work you can accomplish with the same expenditure of energy.

Your heart, like any other muscle, tends to lose strength and tone when it is not regularly exercised with sufficient intensity. The rate at which this loss occurs depends upon a number of factors, including the way you eat, how you handle stress, your use of tobacco and alcohol, as well as your basic genetic make-up.

On the other hand, the health and efficiency of your cardio-respiratory system can be maintained and increased by making improvements in these areas, and by a program of regular aerobic activity (aerobic means "with oxygen").

Aerobic exercise elevates your heart rate to between 60 and 80 percent of its maximum for your age, and keeps it there for at least 15 minutes, and preferably for 30 minutes or more, at a time (see table on page 22).

When significant weight loss is an objective, the greatest benefits are likely to be achieved by extending the duration of your exercise session to between 30 and 60 minutes. At the outset, this may necessitate an exercise heart rate that is at the lower end of the recommended range—perhaps 60 percent of your age adjusted maximum. For many overweight people, long vigorous walks are the preferred form of physical activity.

Ideally aerobic activity is accomplished every day—three days per week is a minimum. Because aerobic conditioning deteriorates relatively quickly with inactivity, it's best not to allow two days to go by without an aerobic workout.

Your aerobic exercise may consist of walking, jogging, running, jumping rope, trampolining, bicycling, skating, swimming, rowing, dancercise, cross-country skiing, or possibly courtsports—any vigorous activity that is sufficiently continuous to maintain your desired exercise heart rate. Activities which involve a lot of starting and stopping usually don't work for this purpose.

THE FIVE PRINCIPLES OF A SAFE AND EFFECTIVE EXERCISE PROGRAM

I. Range	Muscle & Joint Flexibility	Cardio-Respiratory Capacity	Muscle/Bone Balance & Strength
II. Intensity	Execute a full range of possible motions for each of your major joints and muscles.	Engage in continuous activity at your age-adjusted target heart rate.	Selectively exert each of your major muscles.
III. Duration	15 to 30 seconds per movement (9-12 minutes total).	Build from 10 minutes or less to at least 1/2 hour.	8 to 12 repetitions per muscle group (15-20 minutes total).
IV. Frequency	Not less than once a day.	Daily if possible, and not less than every other day.	Every other day, or not less than twice a week.
V. Progression	Extend your range of motion as your flexibility increases.	Gradually intensify your activity while maintaining your target heart rate.	Increase resistance as your strength develops.

A fully effective exercise program activates all three of these distinct physical potentials.

One of the first steps to take in getting started in your exercise program is obtaining the proper equipment. A good pair of running shoes, for example, is essential to creating an enjoyable experience and protecting yourself from possible injury.

As an aside, many people enjoy working out with a friend. Sometimes it's difficult to do this while maintaining the proper exercise intensity. Make certain that you are not attempting to maintain someone else's pace. If necessary, go your own way during your workout, and get together again later. Any competition that may be associated with your program should be light and friendly, contributing only to your enjoyment and motivation for more.

In a well designed cardio-respiratory exercise program, each session includes five essential steps:

Step 1: Pre-exercise stretch

To minimize your risk of pulling a muscle, begin your aerobic workout with a few simple stretches as shown on pages 26, 27 and 28.

Step 2: Warm-up

Following your stretches, and prior to your full-blown exercise, give yourself 5 minutes of cardio-vascular warm-up, performing the same activity you will use for your more vigorous workout. Warm-up is important to open the arterial pathways in your heart and in the other muscles which you will be using. It should be vigorous enough to produce a heart rate approximately 10 to 20 beats per minute slower than your full exercise rate.

Step 3: Aerobic workout

Following your warm-up, bring the intensity of your exercise up to a level that sustains your intended heart rate. In the beginning, keep your heart rate at the low end of the target training range—65 to 70% of your age-adjusted maximum heart rate. If this level feels like too much of an exertion for you, begin even lower, perhaps at 60%, and stay at that level for the first two weeks. Then increase it to 65% for a week, then to 70% for a week, and so on until you can comfortably maintain 75 to 80% of your maximum. There's no need to rush. Your exercise should never be painful. With easy progression, you'll soon be safely back in good condition.

At first the duration of your workout may be short—perhaps only 3 to 5 minutes. As you build your endurance you'll be able to lengthen your workout to 12, 20, then 30 minutes or more. Ideally your daily aerobic workout will be performed at your training heart rate for 20 to 60 minutes.

Step 4: Cool-down

One of the benefits of vigorous activity is that it distributes your blood supply widely throughout your body, bathing all of your cells in life-giving energy. During this time, the circulation of blood—particularly its return to your heart—is assisted by the motion of your muscles. If you were to stop your activity abruptly, your heart might be momentary unable to handle the circulation on its own, and "blood pooling" may occur. This can result in mild shock, hyperventilation or muscle cramping. A 5 minute cool-down of slower paced activity will allow your heart to safely return to its usual rate.

Step 5: Post-exercise stretch

After vigorous physical activity, the muscles which have been used will naturally tend to contract. You can normalize your muscles while they are still warm from the activity by performing a brief set of post-exercise stretches. Without proper stretching, aerobic activity—which often uses the rear thigh and lower back

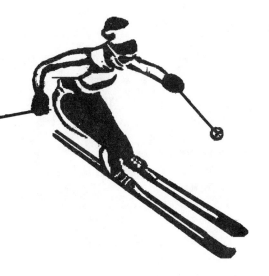

Many activities which are quite demanding physically—such as cross country skiing—are enjoyed by large numbers of people every year. Yet not all activities are suitable for everyone. Choose for yourself those activities that are appropriate to your physical condition, and that take advantage of your natural environment.

Take proper precautions

Please be sure to observe this precautionary note taken from guidelines provided by the National Heart, Lung & Blood Institute: If you are not accustomed to vigorous exercise, and if any of these conditions apply to you, talk with your physician before starting your exercise program:

- Heart trouble, heart murmur, or previous heart attack.
- Frequent pains or pressure, when exercising, in the left or mid-chest area, left neck, shoulder or arm.
- Frequent faintness or dizziness.
- Extreme breathlessness after mild exertion.
- Uncontrolled high blood pressure or unknown blood pressure.
- Bone or joint problems such as arthritis.
- Age over 60.
- Family history of premature coronary artery disease.
- Any other health condition which might need special attention when exercising (for example, insulin-dependent diabetes).

muscles—can produce an abnormal pelvic tilt accompanied by low back pain. Performing the post-exercise stretches specified on page 27 and 28 will help you to avoid such potential problems.

Your target heart rate

To assure that you are maintaining the correct exercise intensity, you must be able to monitor your heart rate during exercise. Heart rate is best determined by placing the second and third fingers along the thumb side of the opposite wrist, and counting the pulsations for ten seconds.

While exercising, stop periodically and take a ten-second count. It is important to quickly determine your exercise heart rate before the slower recovery rate commences. If you find that your heart rate is below the rate you have selected for your workout, increase the speed or intensity of your activity. Then, after a minute or so, take another count and adjust your intensity accordingly. If your heart rate is above your intended rate, continue your exercise, reducing the intensity a bit until you are maintaining the desired rate.

A note about exceeding the target rate: it may seem that if 75% of your maximum is good, then 90% might be even better. This is not generally the case. Above 80% of the maximum rate for your age, your activity may become "anaerobic"— that is, your body may not be able to supply sufficient oxygen to sustain the activity, resulting in early exhaustion. Aerobic activity is accomplished at a level which can be maintained for an extended period, once you are in reasonably good condition. Sprinting and weight lifting are anaerobic activities in that they intentionally press the body to the limits of its capability over a short span of time. While these are properly used to build speed, agility, strength and muscle mass, by themselves they do not provide an adequate cardio-vascular workout.

When you're ready to participate in two of the three types of recommended activities, add a complete five-part cardio-respiratory workout to your daily full-body stretches. Engaging in an aerobic workout once each day is ideal, while every other day is adequate. By performing your full-body stretches just prior to your aerobic activity, they can serve as the first part of your aerobic workout— the pre-exercise stretch.

Select aerobic activities that you'll enjoy, such as swimming, bicycling, jogging, walking, rowing, dancercise or basketball. It's not necessary that the activity be the same each day. For example, you may enjoy playing a game of racquetball two or three times a week. While this is an excellent form of physical activity, it may not provide you with a complete aerobic workout in your target training range. However, when performed in combination with a more aerobic activity— such as swimming—on the off-days, the two can work together to keep you in great shape with a high level of enjoyment.

After you have decided which aerobic activities you'd like to perform, determine where and when you are going to accomplish them. Be specific, considering how to fit them into your schedule, and allowing sufficient time for a shower afterwards as well as any necessary travel. To complete all five parts of your aerobic workout, set aside at least 25 minutes at the outset, gradually building up to 45 minutes or more per session. Make the appropriate entries in your Planning Calendar (page 4) to represent your aerobic activities. Make sure that you obtain any necessary equipment well in advance of your first scheduled session.

Whatever you do, **don't allow yourself to overdo it.** This is a common tendency during the first few times out, when you may be inclined to expect your performance to be at the same level as you may have experienced years ago. To get a realistic idea of how to proceed, review the easy progressions outlined in

Target Training Heart Rate varies from person to person. You can use this formula, provided by the American College of Sports Medicine, to determine your personal training range.

	TRAINING RANGE	
	low end	high end
Start with this number	220	220
Minus your present age	-_____	-_____
Equals maximum rate	=_____	=_____
Minus resting heart rate	-_____	-_____
Equals maximum reserve	=_____	=_____
Multiplied by (percent)	X _.6_	X _.8_
Equals target reserve rate	=_____	=_____
Plus resting heart rate	+_____	+_____
Equals **your training rate**	=_____	=_____
Divided by 6	+_____ 6	+_____ 6
Equals **10 second rate**	=_____	=_____

*Measure your resting heart rate before getting out of bed in the morning. Take your pulse for 10 seconds. Multiply this ten-second count by 6 to arrive at your one-minute resting heart rate.

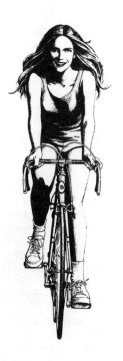

the walking and jogging programs provided on page 25. Once again, patient determination and persistence are your greatest assets for living well, while impatience and procrastination are ever-threatening thieves of the success that you deserve, and that you can surely achieve.

Muscle/Bone Balance, Tone and Strength

The third component of an effective physical activity program is body toning, which develops the **strength, symmetry and balance of your muscle and bone structure.** For most people, this kind of exercise is not intended to build "bulging" muscles, although you can certainly use it to add muscle mass wherever you would like. Rather, it is designed to **improve your tone and prevent the reduction of bone density and muscle mass** which tends to occur when your strength is not used.

Without a balanced combination of proper nutrients and regular activity, significant loss of bone may begin at about age 30 for women, and age 50 for men. With passing years of inactivity, the bones may gradually weaken, resulting in poor posture ("dowager's hump"), a loss of physical stature, and increased risk of breakage. In addition to exercise, an adequate intake of calcium is essential to maintaining bone density.

You can maintain your body tone in just 2 or 3 short sessions per week of 15 to 20 minutes each. The methods which may be used include a variety of workout machines, free weights, isometrics (muscle on muscle resistance), calisthenics and slimnastics. An easily executed set of body toning exercises which require no special equipment are given on pages 30 and 31.

When your stretching and aerobic programs are firmly in place, you're ready to begin your body toning activity. Body toning is effective when performed two or three times each week in addition to your daily stretching and aerobic activities. Precede your body toning workouts with full-body stretches and follow them up with the brief set of post-exercise stretches. You can tone all of your major muscles—thighs (front and back), calves, stomach, waist, chest, shoulders, back and arms—in just 15 to 20 minutes per session. Enter your body toning periods into your Planning Calendar on page 4.

As a general rule, if you're short of time one day, choose first to do your stretches and aerobic workout. The benefits are more fundamental and immediate, and these capacities tend to diminish more rapidly when they are not adequately utilized.

First plan, and then track your daily activity

Use your Planning Calendar (page 4) and Daily Performance Record (page 60) to help establish and maintain an optimal program of regular physical activity. At this point you may want to take another look at your Planning Calendar to make certain that everything you have planned fits well into your schedule. These items appear in the Performance Record for your review each day:

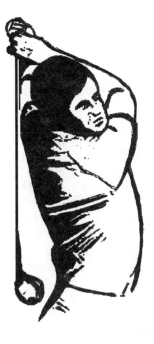

Many popular activities which serve as valuable sources of relaxation may offer few physical benefits unless they are properly performed. Golf, for example, is an excellent exercise when the course is briskly walked rather than driven in a motorized cart.

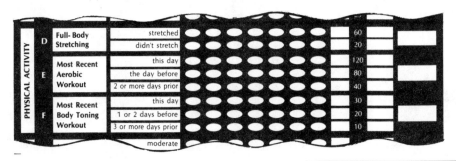

CALORIE EXPENDITURE CHART

Activity raises the body heat, or metabolic rate. This elevated body heat burns off calories not only during the period of activity itself, but also for several hours afterwards. This chart gives a rough approximation of the calories expended in selected activities by a person weighing 150 pounds. Proportionally more will be expended for additional body weight, and less for lower body weight.

Activity	Calories Per Minute
Dancing —	
Ballroom	5.4
Dancercise	7.0
Disco	6.5
Slow	4.4
Square or round	6.0
Gardening —	
General	3.8
Lawn mowing (hand mower)	7.7
Planting seedlings	4.8
Raking	5.4
General Activities —	
Driving a car	2.8
Eating	1.7
Lying at ease	1.5
Sex	7.2
Sitting quietly	1.7
Sleeping (basal metabolism)	1.0
Standing quietly	1.7
Walking — 17 min./mile	5.4
Housekeeping Tasks —	
Bed-making	3.9
Carpet cleaning	3.5
Cooking	3.5
Food Shopping	4.5
Ironing	2.7
Knitting/Sewing	1.8
Mopping floor	4.8
Scrubbing floors (vigorously)	12.0
Occupational Activity —	
Bricklaying	4.0
Carpentry	6.8
Desk work — general	2.2
typing	1.8
Farm work in field	7.3
Painting at an easel	2.0
Piano playing	3.2
Sports/Athletics —	
Archery	2.8
Badminton — singles	5.6
Basketball — full court	12.0
half court	5.0
Bowling	3.5

Activity	Calories Per Minute
Sports/Athletics (continued) —	
Calisthenics	5.2
Canoeing — 15 min./mile	6.9
Circuit training	5.5
Cycling — 5 min./mile	10.6
casual	4.6
Golf — foursome carrying clubs	6.0
walking without clubs	4.6
with cart	3.4
Gymnastics	5.2
Handball	10.9
Hiking — without load	5.0
with 40 lb. backpack	6.8
climbing without load	9.5
climbing with 10 lb. load	10.1
Horseback riding — trot	8.0
walk	4.0
Interval training	10.8
Judo/karate	5.2
Mountain climbing	9.5
Racquetball	10.0
Roller skating — speed	11.2
casual	5.8
Rope-skipping — 80 turns/min.	13.3
Running — 6 min./mile	16.2
jogging 8 min./mile	12.6
Skating — high speed	15.0
casual	5.8
Skiing — cross country	11.6
down-hill (vigorously)	9.5
Skin diving	10.0
Soccer	12.0
Softball or baseball	4.7
Squash	10.7
Surfing	9.2
Swimming — 50 yds./min.	10.5
casual	5.3
Tennis — singles	6.0
doubles	4.6
table tennis	4.0
Trampolining	5.6
Volleyball — 2 players	9.2
6 players	5.8
Water skiing	7.8
Weight training	7.8

CARDIO-RESPIRATORY EXERCISE PROGRAMS

A WALKING PROGRAM

	Warm Up	Target Zone Exercise	Cool Down	Total Time
Week 1	Walk slowly 5 min.	Walk briskly 5 min.	Walk slowly 5 min.	15 min.
Week 2	Walk slowly 5 min.	Walk briskly 7 min.	Walk slowly 5 min.	17 min.
Week 3	Walk slowly 5 min.	Walk briskly 9 min.	Walk slowly 5 min.	19 min.
Week 4	Walk slowly 5 min.	Walk briskly 11 min.	Walk slowly 5 min.	21 min.
Week 5	Walk slowly 5 min.	Walk briskly 13 min.	Walk slowly 5 min.	23 min.
Week 6	Walk slowly 5 min.	Walk briskly 15 min.	Walk slowly 5 min.	25 min.
Week 7	Walk slowly 5 min.	Walk briskly 18 min.	Walk slowly 5 min.	28 min.
Week 8	Walk slowly 5 min.	Walk briskly 20 min.	Walk slowly 5 min.	30 min.
Week 9	Walk slowly 5 min.	Walk briskly 23 min.	Walk slowly 5 min.	33 min.
Week 10	Walk slowly 5 min.	Walk briskly 26 min.	Walk slowly 5 min.	36 min.
Week 11	Walk slowly 5 min.	Walk briskly 28 min.	Walk slowly 5 min.	38 min.
Week 12	Walk slowly 5 min.	Walk briskly 30 min.	Walk slowly 5 min.	40 min.

Week 13 on:

Check your pulse periodically to be sure you are exercising within your target zone. As you get more in shape, try exercising within the upper range of your heart zone. Remember to enjoy yourself.

If you are over 40 and have not been active, begin with the walking program. After completing the walking program, you can start with week 3 of the jogging program.

A JOGGING PROGRAM

	WARM UP	TARGET ZONE EXERCISING	COOL DOWN	TOTAL TIME
Week 1	Stretch 5 min.	Walk 10 min.	Walk slowly 3 min., stretch 2 min.	20 min.
Week 2	Stretch 5 min., walk 5 min.	Jog 1 min., walk 5 min., jog 1 min.	Walk slowly 3 min., stretch 2 min.	22 min.
Week 3	Stretch 5 min., walk 5 min.	Jog 3 min., walk 5 min., jog 3 min.	Walk slowly 3 min., stretch 2 min.	26 min.
Week 4	Stretch 5 min., walk 4 min.	Jog 5 min., walk 4 min., jog 5 min.	Walk slowly 3 min., stretch 2 min.	28 min.
Week 5	Stretch 5 min., walk 4 min.	Jog 5 min., walk 4 min., jog 5 min.	Walk slowly 3 min., stretch 2 min.	28 min.
Week 6	Stretch 5 min., walk 4 min.	Jog 6 min., walk 4 min., jog 6 min.	Walk slowly 3 min., stretch 2 min.	30 min.
Week 7	Stretch 5 min., walk 4 min.	Jog 7 min., walk 4 min., jog 7 min.	Walk slowly 3 min., stretch 2 min.	32 min.
Week 8	Stretch 5 min., walk 4 min.	Jog 8 min., walk 4 min., jog 8 min.	Walk slowly 3 min., stretch 2 min.	34 min.
Week 9	Stretch 5 min., walk 4 min.	Jog 9 min., walk 4 min., jog 9 min.	Walk slowly 3 min., stretch 2 min.	36 min.
Week 10	Stretch 5 min., walk 4 min.	Jog 13 min.	Walk slowly 3 min., stretch 2 min.	27 min.
Week 11	Stretch 5 min., walk 4 min.	Jog 15 min.	Walk slowly 3 min., stretch 2 min.	29 min.
Week 12	Stretch 5 min., walk 4 min.	Jog 17 min.	Walk slowly 3 min., stretch 2 min.	31 min.
Week 13	Stretch 5 min., walk 2 min., jog slowly 2 min.	Jog 17 min.	Walk slowly 3 min., stretch 2 min.	31 min.
Week 14	Stretch 5 min., walk 1 min., jog slowly 3 min.	Jog 17 min.	Walk slowly 3 min., stretch 2 min.	31 min.
Week 15	Stretch 5 min., jog slowly 3 min.	Jog 17 min.	Walk slowly 3 min., stretch 2 min.	30 min.

Week 16 on:

Check your pulse periodically to see if you are exercising within your target zone. As you become more fit, try exercising within the upper range of your target zone. Remember that your goal is to continue to get the benefits you are seeking, while enjoying your activity. Listen to your body and build up less quickly, if needed.

FULL BODY STRETCHES

Frequent stretching, besides simply feeling good, helps you maintain the flexibility of your muscles, and the range of motion of your joints.

When performing your stretches, observe these guidelines:
- Once a day, perform each stretch for 15 to 30 seconds. The entire sequence takes less than 12 minutes.
- Stretch slowly and gently, never bouncing or forcing the movement.
- Breathe fully and naturally — at a normal rate — relaxing a little further into your stretch with each exhalation.

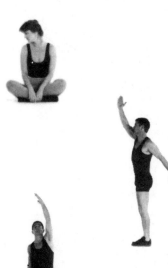

NECK STRETCHES

While either standing or sitting, relax your neck, allowing your head to drop gently forward. Slowly turn and lift your head until you are facing to one side; then slowly rotate back down to the center. Repeat, turning and lifting your head to the other side, and then back down. Repeat 5 times.

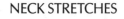

ARM CIRCLES

While standing, slowly rotate and stretch your arms for 10 seconds as in the backstroke; then reverse the direction of rotation for another 10 seconds.

REACH-UP STRETCH

While standing or sitting, stretch and reach toward the ceiling; first with your right arm, then with your left, alternating for 10 times.

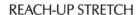

SIDE STRETCH

While standing or sitting, with your hands clasped above your head, first bend gently to the left and hold for 5 seconds; then repeat to the right. Repeat 6 times.

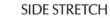

SHOULDER, TRICEPS AND UPPER BACK STRETCH

While sitting or standing, gently pull your elbow across your chest toward your opposite shoulder. Hold for 10 seconds. Repeat with other arm.

Sit or stand with one arm stretched upward and bent at the elbow so the hand is behind your head. With the other hand, slowly and gently pull the elbow toward a position behind your head. Repeat with other arm.

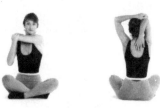

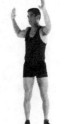

WAIST TWIST

While standing with your legs bent slightly and your upper arms raised to shoulder height, gently twist your upper body from side to side while keeping your lower body stationary. Continue for 10 twists to each side.

LEG STRETCH

Assuming a sprinter's position, stretch your achilles tendons and calf muscles by pointing your back heel while slowly lowering your hips. Hold for 10 seconds. Repeat with your other leg.

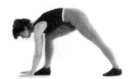

HIP AND THIGH STRETCH

While leaning forward on your fingertips, one leg extended back with its knee resting on the floor, the other leg forward so its knee is directly over its ankle, lower the front of your hip downward for an easy stretch. Hold for 30 seconds. Repeat with other leg.

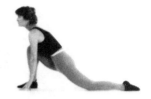

LEG, GROIN AND BACK STRETCH

Squat down with your feet flat, your toes pointed outward at a slight angle, your heels 4-12 inches apart (depending upon your flexibility), your knees to the outside of your shoulders and your shoulders directly above your big toes. If you wish, you may lean against a wall for balance. Hold a comfortable stretch for 30 seconds.

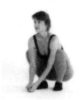

TRUNK FLEXION*

While sitting with your legs extended and your feet flexed, reach for your toes. Bend forward gently from your hips while keeping your back straight. Hold for 10 seconds. Repeat 5 times.

ANKLE PULL*

While sitting with your knees bent, your heels on the floor and your hands grasping your toes, slowly straighten one leg until fully extended, pulling back on the toes. Hold this position for 5 seconds.

After returning the straightened leg to a bent position, extend the other leg, and hold it there for 5 seconds. Repeat for 1 to 3 minutes.

Next, perform the same exercise while grasping the outside of the foot near the toes. And finally, repeat the exercise while grasping the inside border of the foot near the toes.

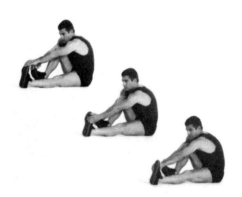

HAMSTRING, GROIN AND BACK STRETCH

Sitting on the floor with your legs outstretched and spread wide in front, keep your chin in and your back straight while slowly bending forward from the hips toward the foot of one leg. Hold for 30 seconds. Repeat, bending toward the foot of your other leg, and then finally bending toward the middle.

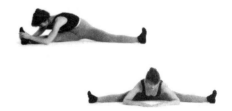

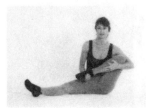

ANKLE, FOOT AND TOE STRETCHES

While sitting on the floor with your legs outstretched, hold your right leg in front of you by supporting it with your right hand. With your left hand, rotate your ankle 10 times clockwise and 10 times counter-clockwise through a complete range of motion. Next gently pull the toes toward you with your fingers. Hold for 10 seconds, and repeat. Repeat with your left leg.

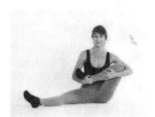

UPPER HAMSTRING AND HIP STRETCHES

While in the same sitting position, hold your ankle with one hand and your knee with the other. Give the upper back part of your leg an easy stretch by gently pulling the entire leg toward your chest. *Move your leg as a single unit to avoid stressing the knee.* Hold for 20 seconds and repeat. Repeat with other leg.

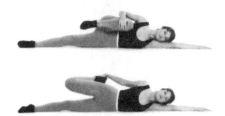

BUTTOCK STRETCH*

While lying on your side with your legs straight, pull your top knee toward your chest and hold it there for 10 seconds. Relaxing the tension, slide your hand to your ankle, and then pull your ankle toward the rear, stretching the front of your upper leg. Hold this position for 10 seconds, then relax. Repeat the entire sequence 5 times. Turn to the other side and repeat with other leg.

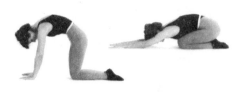

MAD CAT

While on hands and knees, exhale as you arch your spine as high as possible, pulling your chin toward your chest — hold for 5 seconds and then relax. Repeat 5 times. Finish by sitting backwards onto your calves, leaving your arms outstretched on the floor above your head.

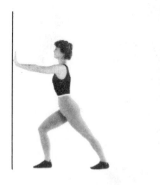

ACHILLES TENDON STRETCH*

Standing 3 to 4 feet from a wall with your hands pressed against it, extend one of your legs back 3 to 4 additional feet. Keep your back heel in contact with the floor while slowly moving your trunk toward the wall by bending your front knee. Without bouncing, give your rear leg muscles a good stretch for 5 seconds, then repeat with the other leg. Continue with this for 1 to 3 minutes.

---

* **After aerobic or body toning exercise, stretch out your rear thigh and lower back muscles with these post-exercise stretches. Then finish off with a set of Sit-Ups as shown on page 25.**

Special Exercises for Flat Feet

If you have flat feet, you may benefit from including these exercises in your daily stretching routine. Wearing orthotics may also help — these are special arch supports available from a podiatrist.

MARBLE PICK-UP

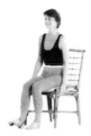

Sit barefoot in a chair with a few wads of paper the size of large marbles on the floor in front of you. Forcefully grip one of the paper balls with the toes of your right foot, pick it up, and hold it for 5 seconds. Repeat with your left foot. Continue for 1 to 3 minutes.

TOWEL PULL

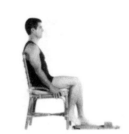

Place a towel with a 2 to 5 pound weight on it on the floor in front of your chair. Sitting barefoot, grip the towel with the toes of one foot, and pull it completely past the heel of your other foot. Change feet and repeat.

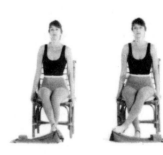

Next place the towel and weight to the right of your feet. Gripping the towel with the toes of your right foot, move it completely past your left foot. Repeat using your left foot.

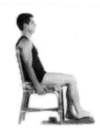

And finally, place the towel and weight behind your heels. Using each foot in turn, grip the towel and move it forward past the toes of the other foot.

BODY TONING

Body toning exercises develop the tone, strength, symmetry and balance of your muscle and bone structure. The methods which may be used include isometrics, slimnastics, a variety of exercise machines, and free weights.

When performing your body toning exercises, follow these guidelines:
- Prepare yourself by performing the full-body stretches provided in the previous section.
- Execute each body toning exercise smoothly and rhythmically. Maintain good form at all times.
- During the exercises, inhale at the time of least exertion; exhale at the time of greatest exertion.
- After you have completed your body toning exercises, finish up with a brief stretch, using the post exercise stretches specified on pages 20-23.

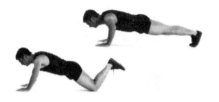

PUSH-UPS

Begin by lying on your stomach with your hands shoulder width apart. Keeping your body rigid, push up until your arms are straight. Then, by bending at the elbows, lower your body until you can touch your chin to the floor. Repeat 5-30 times. If this is too difficult, keep your knees on the floor while performing the exercise.

HIP RAISE

Lying on your back with your hands at your sides and your knees bent, push up, tighten and hold your hips and buttocks for 5-10 seconds, then lower. Repeat 5-15 times.

SIDE LEG LIFTS

While lying on your side with your legs straight, lift the top leg as high as you can and hold for 2 seconds before lowering. Repeat 6-20 times.

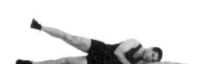

Repeat the same exercise, *this time pointing the toes of your top foot.* On each downswing, lower your pointed toes behind the heel of your stationary leg without actually touching the floor.

Repeat the same exercise once again, *this time flexing your top foot* (opposite of pointing). On each downswing, lower your heel to a point in front of your stationary ankle without touching it to the floor.

Turn over and repeat the entire sequence with your other leg.

INNER-THIGH RAISE

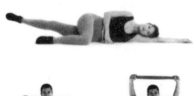

Lie on your side with head resting on your extended arm, bottom leg extended and foot flexed, top leg bent and resting on floor. While keeping your hips rolled forward and your lower knee facing forward, lift bottom leg — squeezing your inner thigh — then lower it again. Without touching your leg to the floor between lifts, repeat 6-20 times with each leg.

TOWEL STRETCH

Grasping towel ends, simultaneously extend and flex your arms and shoulders. Use a variety of positions, including above, behind and in front of your head.

PUSH AND PULL

With your hands opposing each other at chest level, press palms together for 5-10 seconds. Repeat several times. Then grasp your hands or wrists at chest level and pull for 5-10 seconds. Repeat several times.

NECK ISOMETRICS

With your hands on your forehead, keep your neck straight while pushing with slowly increasing pressure until firm neck tension is reached. Hold for 5 seconds. Repeat with hands on back of head. Repeat with one hand on side of head. Repeat with other hand on opposite side of head.

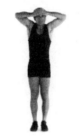 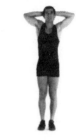

HALF SQUATS

Standing with your hands on your hips, lower your body to a half squat position while thrusting your arms forward, then return to the starting position. Repeat 5-20 times.

Standing with your feet turned outward, lower your body to a half squat while raising your arms sideways, then return to the starting position. Repeat 5 to 20 times.

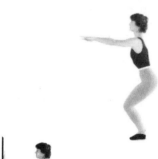

CALF RAISES

Using a wall or chair for balance, stand with feet together and one leg lifted slightly. Raise and lower opposite heel 20-50 times. Repeat with other leg.

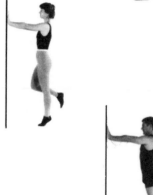

FULL LEG & BUTTOCK TIGHTENING

Standing with hands on wall for balance, raise both heels while tightening calves, thighs and buttocks. Hold 10 seconds; relax 10 seconds; and repeat.

SIT-UPS

Lie flat on your back with knees bent at 45 degrees, arms crossed on chest and stomach muscles pulled in tightly. Curl up and forward until your shoulders are lifted 5 to 6 inches off the floor; then lower. Without relaxing your stomach muscles, curl up and forward again, this time while pointing your left shoulder toward your right knee; then lower. Once again, while continuing to maintain stomach muscle tension, curl up and forward while pointing your right shoulder toward your left knee; then lower.

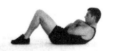

Perform five repetitions of this three step routine to begin with, slowly working up to 20 repetitions (60 total sit-ups). Note that this exercise does not call for curling up to a full sitting position, as this tends to stress the lower back, and does not further strengthen the stomach muscles.

EXERCISES FOR THE LOWER BACK

Seven out of ten adults over the age of 35 suffer from some degree of low back pain, much of it due to two controllable factors: insufficient trunk flexibility and weak abdominal muscles. An imbalance of strength or length between the abdominal muscles and the rear thigh and back muscles may cause an improper pelvic tilt, thus producing a misalignment of the spine with low grade irritation and pain. This condition sometimes occurs when the legs are rapidly strengthened without complementary stretching exercises.

These exercises shorten and strengthen the abdominal muscles while stretching and lengthening the rear thigh and low back muscles.

The exercises are presented in three parts: beginning, intermediate and advanced. If you are not currently experiencing back pain you may begin the intermediate exercises after about a week of preconditioning with the beginning exercises, later adding the advanced.

If you have been suffering with pain in the lower back, then you may experience minor, short-term discomfort while performing some of the exercises. If it does not persist, and does not bother you during subsequent hours, you may want to continue those exercises. **Discontinue immediately any exercise which produces significant or continuing pain.**

The beginning exercises are relatively passive, promoting moderate stretching and conditioning. For the first three weeks, these exercises may be performed every other day. If no additional pain is experienced, increase the number of exercise sessions to 4 or 5 days per week for the next three weeks, and to 6 or 7 days per week for the following three weeks. After the ninth week, many people perform the exercises twice each day.

If you have no additional pain following the end of the twelfth week, continue the beginning exercises while carefully adding the intermediate. After several weeks of performing the intermediate exercises, you may add the advanced.

Execute each exercise slowly and gently for at least one minute.

Beginning Exercises

BACK PRESS (legs straight)

While lying flat on your back with your legs straight, tighten your buttocks muscles, pull your stomach muscles in tightly, and then press your lower spine to the floor. Hold this for ten seconds, then relax for ten seconds. Repeat this sequence three or more times.

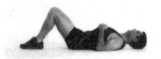

BACK PRESS (knees bent)

Still lying flat on your back, perform three or more additional back presses while your knees are bent at a 45 degree angle.

Lower back pain — a troublesome by-product of sedentary living — is experienced by seven out of ten adults over the age of 35. As much as 80 percent of all back pain is related to two controllable factors: trunk flexibility and abdominal strength.

KNEE TO CHEST

Lying flat on your back with your legs straight, pull your stomach muscles in tightly while slowly bringing one knee up towards your chest. Grasp the front of the leg with both hands, pulling it to your chest. After holding this for 5 seconds, release the leg and straighten it. Do the same with the other leg, and then repeat several times.

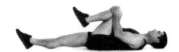

FORWARD SPINE CURL

Lie flat on your back with your knees bent at 45 degrees and your arms across your chest. While tightening your stomach muscles and keeping your lower spine and pelvis in contact with the floor, slowly curl your head forward until your chin comfortably touches your chest, then continue until your shoulders are lifted 5-6 inches off the floor. Hold this for 5 seconds before returning to the starting position. Repeat several times.

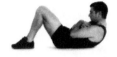

MAD CAT

While on hands and knees, exhale as you arch your spine as high as possible, pulling your chin toward your chest — hold for 5 seconds, then relax and repeat.

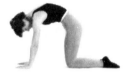

FORWARD LEAN

Sit on the floor with your knees bent to the sides, the bottoms of your feet touching each other, and your hands grasping your feet. With your stomach muscles tightened, slowly bend forward, move your face toward your feet as far as you comfortably can. After holding this for 10 seconds, return to the starting position and repeat.

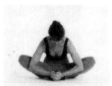

FORWARD TRUNK LEAN

Sit on the floor with your legs straight and your hands grasping the backs of your knees. With your stomach muscles tightened, slowly lean forward, bringing your face toward your knees as far as is comfortable. After holding this for 10 to 30 seconds, return to the starting position and repeat.

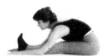

Intermediate Exercises

BUTTOCK STRETCH

While lying on your side with your legs straight, pull your top knee toward your chest and hold it there for 10 seconds. Relaxing the tension, slide your hand to your ankle, and then pull your ankle toward the rear, stretching the front of your upper leg. Hold this position for 10 seconds, then relax and repeat the entire sequence. Turn to the other side and repeat with other leg.

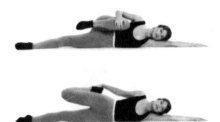

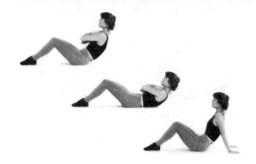

SIT-BACK

On a padded surface, sit with your knees bent at a 45 degree angle and your hands folded in front of your chest. While pulling your stomach muscles in tightly, slowly lean back until your shoulders touch the floor (this movement should take 4-6 seconds to complete). With the assistance of your hands and elbows, return to the starting position and repeat two or more times.

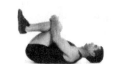

KNEES TO CHEST

Lie on your back with your knees bent at a 45 degree angle, your arms at your sides, and your hands flat on the floor. While pulling your stomach muscles in tightly, slowly bring both knees toward your chest. Continuing the motion, grasp your knees with your hands and pull them toward your chest. Hold this position for 5 seconds before returning to the starting position. Rest for 5 seconds and repeat three or more times.

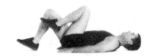

ALTERNATE KNEES TO CHEST

Lie on your back with your knees bent at a 45 degree angle, and your spine pressed to the floor. With your stomach muscles pulled in tightly, slowly bring one knee to your chest. Then, while returning the first leg to its starting position, simultaneously bring the other knee to your chest. Continue bringing alternate knees to your chest for 30 seconds, each time briefly touching the heel of the down foot to the floor.

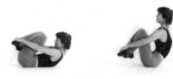

BACK ROLL

On a padded floor, lie on your back with your knees bent to your chest, your ankles crossed, and your hands clasping your ankles. With your stomach muscles pulled in tightly, begin rocking by curling your head forward while pulling down on your ankles. Gently rock forward and backward 5-10 times, ending in a sitting position. Rest for 5 seconds, and then repeat.

Advanced Exercises

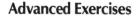

STRAIGHT LEG PULL

While sitting with your knees bent, your heels on the floor and your hands grasping your toes, slowly straighten one leg until fully extended, pulling back on the toes — hold for 15 seconds. After returning the straightened leg to a bent position, straighten the other leg and hold for 15 seconds. Repeat one or more times.

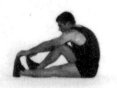

ISOMETRIC SIT-UP

On a padded surface, balance on your buttocks with your legs and spine straight, and your feet and shoulders raised off the floor. While your stomach muscles are pulled in tightly, lean forward at the waist, simultaneously bending your knees and bringing them toward your face. Hold this position for 5 seconds, then return to the starting position. Repeat several times.

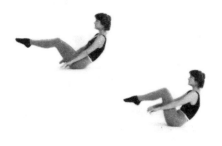

OPPOSITE KNEE SIT-UP

Lie on your back with your knees bent at a 45 degree angle and your hands touching the sides of your head. With your stomach muscles pulled in tightly, curl upwards with your head and shoulders, simultaneously bringing your right knee up to touch your left elbow. Return to the starting position and then repeat, this time touching your left knee to your right elbow. Repeat this alternating sequence several times.

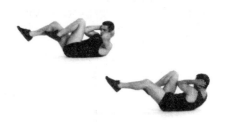

SIDE TILTS

Lie on your back with your arms out to the side on the floor, your legs together, your knees bent at a 45 degree angle, your stomach muscles pulled in tightly, and your feet held 3-5 inches above the floor. While keeping your shoulders, arms and buttocks flat on the floor, tilt your knees to the left side and hold for 5 seconds. After returning to the starting position, tilt your knees to the right side. Repeat several times.

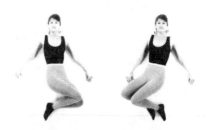

BENT KNEE SHOULDER PULL-UP

Lie on your back with your knees bent, your feet widely separated on the floor, and your hands grasping your shoulders near the neck. With your stomach muscles tightened, curl upwards — first with your head and then with your shoulders, pointing your right elbow toward your left thigh. Hold this position for 15 seconds, then return to the starting position and rest for 10 seconds. Do another pull-up, this time pointing your left elbow toward your right thigh. Repeat the entire sequence one or more times.

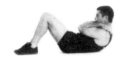

In addition to depending upon stress management and a well designed program of physical activity, your continuing wellness is maintained by proper nutrition. Your body needs certain essential nutrients—carbohydrates, protein, fats, vitamins, minerals, water and air. And it needs them in proper quantity, purity and balance to maintain optimal health and well-being.

The primary vehicles for delivering energy and nutrients to your body are: **protein,** mainly from meats, fish and certain vegetables; **carbohydrates,** primarily from plant food sources; and **fats.** To gain their full benefits, your body needs to receive them in amounts that are closely matched to your requirements: no more and no less.

No single food item can provide you with all the nutrients you need for optimal health. In fact, one of the best ways to assure that you're giving your body everything it needs is to eat a variety of good foods. The greater the variety, the less your chance of either a deficiency or an excess of any single nutrient.

The Basic Food Groups

The easiest and surest way to obtain a balanced variety of good foods is to regularly select from among all the basic food groups. These include:

Carbohydrates

Breads and cereals, including whole grain cereals, rolls, tortillas, noodles, spaghetti, macaroni, pancakes, waffles, muffins, oatmeal, rice, barley, bulgar or cracked wheat.

Leafy green vegetables, including romaine, red and green leaf lettuce, chard, collards and other greens, broccoli, brussel sprouts, cabbage, asparagus, parsley, watercress and scallions.

Fresh fruit and vegetables rich in vitamin C, including citrus fruits, tomatoes, berries, melons, peppers, cabbage, cauliflower, broccoli and brussel sprouts.

Protein

Animal sources, including meats, poultry, seafood and eggs.

Vegetable sources, including dried beans, lentils, split peas, peanuts, peanut butter and other nuts.

Fats

Fats and oils, including butter, margarine, vegetable oils, mayonnaise, salad dressings, cream, seeds, avocadoes, olives and bacon.

Dairy products are a source of carbohydrate, protein and fat, and they are rich in essential vitamins and minerals, especially calcium. However, because in their natural form they are very high in fat, they are best consumed only in skim or low fat form.

Carbohydrates: Quick Energy From Plants

Carbohydrates, chemically the least complex of the major food types, are readily digested into a simple blood sugar called glucose. Glucose fuels your brain activity and other body processes. Your muscles chemically burn glucose, in combination with fat, to release energy for body heat and motion. Carbohydrates also carry many of the vitamins and minerals essential to normal body functioning.

The energy in food is considerable, though its expenditure is not always obvious because it is released gradually and at many points in the body. By way of a comparison, the 375 calorie energy yield of a double dip ice cream cone is equivalent to the explosive power of 1-1/2 sticks of dynamite.

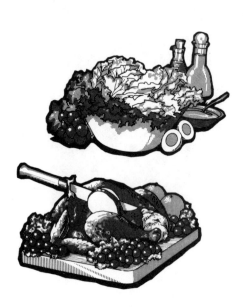

The basic principles of nutrition:

1. Regularly eat a well-balanced variety of unprocessed grains, fresh fruits, vegetables and low-fat dairy products.

2. Eat little meat—3.5 to 4 ounces per serving—and when you do, select those that are low in fat. Remove skin and any visible fats from your meats prior to preparation.

3. Minimize your intake of fats, sugar and salt.

Fiber

Dietary fiber comes from plant food sources only, and consists of that portion of fruits, vegetables, whole grain cereals and other plant foods which is not broken down by the body during digestion. Most unrefined carbohydrates contain fiber which, though undigestible in itself, possesses many positive nutritional qualities. It aids digestion and speeds the elimination of wastes, reducing the concentrations of cancer promoting substances in your intestines. Fiber-rich foods decrease fat absorption, reduce cholesterol in the bloodstream, and stabilize blood sugar levels. Certain plant fibers also help to detoxify various drugs and chemicals. In addition, fiber has the marvelous quality of making you feel full without adding any calories. And finally, fiber helps you to fend off such problems as heart disease, certain types of cancer, diabetes, hemorrhoids and constipation.

Each person's need for fiber is different. While the average person consumes 10 to 20 grams of dietary fiber per day, the recommended amount is 30 to 35 grams. One indicator of whether or not you're eating enough fiber-rich food is your stool: if it's soft and floats, you're more likely to be getting enough fiber; if it's hard and sinks, you could probably use more fibrous foods.

Processed Carbohydrates; Sugar

By removing nutrients and fiber from plant food sources to make products like white flour and sugar, large numbers of calories are concentrated into a low bulk form with little nutritional value, and notable digestive disadvantages. They can be eaten quickly, without producing the sense of fullness normally associated with consuming unprocessed foods having a like number of calories. And they are quickly absorbed into your bloodstream, temporarily flooding your system with more fuel than it needs for efficient operation.

Amazingly, 130 pounds of sugar are consumed per person each year in this country. That's about 36 teaspoons of sugar every day! Much of it comes from packaged foods and soft drinks—a 12-ounce can of soda pop contains about 9 teaspoons of sugar. High sugar intake promotes obesity, diabetes, tooth decay and perhaps even heart disease. You may also experience fatigue after consuming a large amount of sugar in something called reactive hypoglycemia.

There's little doubt that your body works more efficiently when it's not overloaded with sugar. Sugar is more properly used as a seasoning, in small amounts, than it is as a main ingredient in your food.

How to optimize your intake of unrefined carbohydrates:

Step 1. If fresh fruit is not already a regular part of your daily food regimen, concentrate during the first week on adding fruit to your eating patterns. First shop for some good looking fruit—bananas, apples, oranges, grapefruit, peaches, melons, grapes etc.—and then make sure that you have at least one serving of it each day. Fruit makes an excellent snack or dessert, and may be effectively substituted for sweets to help you break the sugar habit.

Step 2. Add fresh raw vegetables daily. While continuing to eat fresh fruit each day, this week add some fresh raw vegetables to your daily food intake. Shop for greens like lettuce, spinach, romaine and parsley. Also pick up such things as carrots, celery, cucumbers, green peppers, cabbage, cauliflower, and tomatoes. Then treat yourself to an attractive, tasty fresh salad each day. And try carrots or celery as a snack in place of sweets.

When evaluating fiber intake, a distinction is made between dietary fiber and crude fiber. Dietary fiber is what remains after human processing in the gastrointestinal tract; whereas crude fiber is what is left over after far more caustic processing as part of a laboratory analysis of the food. For every gram of crude fiber, there may be 2 to 3 grams of dietary fiber. A crude fiber intake of about 6 grams per day is considered ideal.

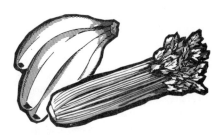

Increasing your intake of fiber is both easy and tasty. Among the foods which contain substantial amounts of fiber are whole grains, such as oats, wheat, rye and barley, as well as fruits and vegetables, legumes. Among the many ways you can increase your intake of fiber are:

- Leave the peel on fruits and vegetables.
- Use brown rice instead of white rice.
- Sprinkle whole grain cereals on casseroles or vegetable dishes for added crunch and fiber.
- Sprinkle granola over fruit or stir into yogurt.
- Eat whole baked or boiled potatoes, including skins, instead of mashed.
- Sauté or stir-fry vegetables. to increase their available fiber content.
- Use unpeeled vegetables in salads, soups, stews and casseroles.
- Leave the peel on fresh fruits .
- Add kidney beans, red beans or other similar beans to soups and stews.
- Use oats in place of flour in crumb-type toppings for fruit crisps and coffeecakes.

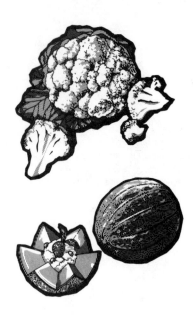

Step 3. Add fresh steamed vegetables. While continuing with your fruit and fresh raw vegetables on a daily basis, this week add fresh (or frozen) steamed vegetables to at least one meal each day. Shop for some broccoli, green beans, peas, corn, carrots, brussel sprouts, cauliflower, cabbage or asparagus—whatever seems good to you. It's better to lightly steam your vegetables than to cook them in water, since this helps to retain the fresh flavor and healthful nutrients.

Step 4. Continue eating raw and steamed vegetables and fresh fruit each day while adding a daily serving of whole grains. Shop for grain products that are not highly processed and that contain as little sugar and preservatives as possible. These products might include breads, dry and cooked cereals, tortillas, rolls or muffins. Even cakes and pie crusts can be made using whole wheat and honey—whole wheat pastry flour is excellent. Try substituting noodles and macaroni made from vegetables and whole grains for those made from highly processed wheat. Use brown rice rather than white. Among the cereals, there are many, both cooked and uncooked, which taste great and contain little or no added sugar or preservatives. Try a variety of grains, including wheat, oats, rice, corn, barley, rye and bulgar or cracked wheat. Oats have recently been shown to be particularly effective in helping to reduce the level of cholesterol in the bloodstream.

Protein: The Body's Building Blocks

Protein is the primary source of building materials for your heart, brain, and other internal organs, as well as for your blood, muscles, skin, hair and nails. Protein also plays an important role in the formation of many essential body chemicals. Your body needs protein, not only for initial growth, but also to replace the billions of cells which die each day and are eliminated.

Over the past century, average protein intake has remained about the same. However, the source of protein has changed. Early in the century, half of the protein came from grains, legumes (peas, beans and lentils), potatoes and other vegetables. The other half came from animal products. Today, a much higher percentage of all the protein consumed comes from animal products. This change toward more animal protein has contributed both to an increase in fat intake and to a decrease in carbohydrate and fiber intake. For example, hamburger is a combination of protein and fat, while pinto beans are a combination of protein, starch and fiber.

If your eating patterns are average, then your protein intake is about twice the amount required to build and repair body tissue. The surplus is either burned as energy or stored as fat. In addition to being associated with fat, animal protein is also a more concentrated source of calories than vegetable protein. So cutting down on animal protein is a natural way to stay slim. It also helps to fortify you against some major problems: heart disease, cancer, high blood pressure, osteoporosis (thinning and weakening of the bones), diverticular disease (an inflammation of the intestines) and kidney stones.

Moderate your intake of protein from animal sources

If you're eating more animal protein than you need, begin cutting down on your portions of meat, substituting potatoes, grains and vegetables. Combining vegetables with grains, legumes or low fat dairy products will enable you to design meatless meals with nourishing good taste which still provide you with a complete protein.

Shop for meats like turkey, chicken and fish instead of high-fat meats such as pork, prime beef, hamburger, duck and lamb. Remove the skin from turkey and chicken prior to cooking. Ground turkey is generally available if you ask your butcher shop for it, and it serves as an excellent substitute for hamburger in virtually all applications.

Excess cholesterol in the blood contributes to the development of fatty deposits in the arteries. Gradually the buildup of these deposits restricts the flow of blood, reducing the volume of oxygen and nutrients that can be supplied to the various parts of the body. This hardening and narrowing of the arteries contributes to many cases of heart attack—which occur when an artery within the heart muscle is blocked, and stroke—which occur when an artery providing blood to the brain is blocked.

Here are some effective strategies that you can use to substantially lower the level of cholesterol in your blood:

- Limit your intake of cholesterol from eggs, red meat, butter and fast foods that have been prepared in animal fat.

- Regularly provide yourself with fish oil, especially from salt water fish such as salmon—that are high in oil.

- Regularly eat oatmeal, especially oat bran.

- Engage in regular exercise.

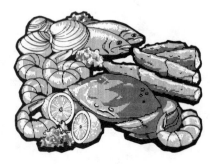

Recent findings suggest that seafood—in particular fish oil—may actually help to counteract some of the more significant health risks associated with excess fat intake. For this reason, regularly eating fish that is high in oil—salmon, for example—is an excellent way of obtaining quality protein.

Fat: Energy, Insulation and Contouring

Fat is a highly concentrated source of energy. The fats in your food are carriers for certain vitamins and aid in the absorption of vitamin D from sunlight. Surplus protein and carbohydrates, as well as excess dietary fats are converted by your liver into body fat for reserve energy. Deposits of fat surround, protect and hold in place your kidneys, liver, heart and other organs, while a layer of subsurface fat helps you to preserve body heat, insulates you from environmental fluctuations, and rounds out the contours of your body. Fat is the primary source of slower burning fuel for body heat and muscular activity.

Fat consumption has been on the rise over the past hundred years, not only because of its presence in sources of animal protein, but also because of a wider availability and use of refined fats and oils, particularly margarines and salad oils. In addition, many of the popular "fast foods" are deep-fried in fat—usually animal fat. Fat is far and away the most concentrated source of calories, so high-fat meals are also high-calorie meals. Further, high-fat meals require more energy to digest, and may leave you with a sleepy, lethargic feeling. They may also produce acid indigestion or "heartburn".

While your body does need a variety of fats daily, you're likely to get most—if not all—of what you need from your protein and carbohydrate sources without having to eat outright fats such as butter, margarine, mayonnaise, salad dressings and oils. In other words, what you eat of these items is essentially for taste and not for nourishment. So it's a good idea to keep your intake of fats to a minimum.

Salt

Although the average person consumes about 5,000 milligrams (mg) of sodium a day, a safe daily intake for adults is considered to be somewhere between 1,100 to 3,000 mg. (One teaspoon of salt contains about 2,000 mg of sodium.) For most people, approximately one-third of sodium intake comes from habitual use of the salt shaker; one-third from processed foods; and one-third as a natural component of food.

Processed foods tend to be both high in sodium and low in the potassium that is ordinarily present in many unprocessed foods. Increased reliance on convenience foods has given rise to a sodium-potassium imbalance which is reflected in a growing incidence of high blood pressure, or hypertension. About one in five adults has high blood pressure, though only about half know it. Unattended, it can lead to arterial disease, heart attack, stroke or kidney failure. You can increase your intake of potassium by eating more fresh fruits, especially bananas, fresh vegetables and potatoes.

Eat Well!

No doubt about it, there's a lot to be said for enjoying nourishing foods that help to keep you well. The rewards are great. And remember, this is not a "don't" routine. Nor is it a "should" routine. This is simply eating intelligently, in a way that fits the realities of living well in the twentieth century.

The payoffs can be relatively immediate: you'll notice an increase in your energy level, shinier hair, clearer skin, and perhaps even a bit more sparkle in your eye. Common discomforts like constipation, heartburn and anemia will decrease or disappear. And over the long haul, your eating patterns will help to promote extraordinary health, longevity and well-being.

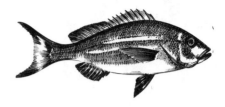

Some ways you can reduce your intake of fats:
- use low fat, or better yet, non-fat dairy products;
- avoid fried foods, including most fast foods;
- use margarine, preferably soft margarine, instead of butter;
- remove visible fat from meat;
- remove skin from turkey and chicken;
- minimize your use of mayonnaise, salad dressings and oils.

Strategies for reducing your intake of salt:
- Remove the salt shaker from the table.
- Read labels carefully to determine the amounts of sodium in processed foods and snacks.
- Moderate your choice of salty foods such as potato chips, pickled foods, cured meats and cheese.
- Prepare more foods "from scratch," reducing or omitting salt.
- Prepare vegetables, pasta, rice and hot cereals with little or no salt.
- Whenever appropriate, accent foods with herbs, spices, onion, garlic, vinegar or citrus fruits instead of salt.

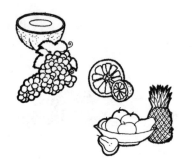

Keep an eye on your progress

Each week you can earn another 210 points in your Living Well program by maintaining healthful eating patterns. Use the Living Well Daily Performance Record (page 60) to keep track of your progress in the three key nutritional areas of carbohydrate intake, fat intake, and eating in moderation.

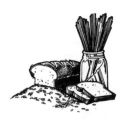

		3 or						
NUTRITIONAL INTAKE	**G**	Amount of Food Eaten	moderate	● ● ● ● ● ● ● ● ● ● ● ●			60	
			a bit too much	● ● ● ● ● ● ● ● ● ● ● ●			40	
			excessive	● ● ● ● ● ● ● ● ● ● ● ●			20	
	H	Intake of Unrefined Carbohydrates	high	● ● ● ● ● ● ● ● ● ● ● ●			75	
			medium	● ● ● ● ● ● ● ● ● ● ● ●			50	
			low	● ● ● ● ● ● ● ● ● ● ● ●			25	
	I	Intake of Fats	low fat	● ● ● ● ● ● ● ● ● ● ● ●			75	
			medium fat	● ● ● ● ● ● ● ● ● ● ● ●			50	
			high fat	● ● ● ● ● ● ● ● ● ● ● ●			25	
			0 or less					

To summarize the information on nutrition, here are some practical guidelines for making sensible daily selections from the four main food groups:

Fruit, raw or steamed vegetables, potato: four servings of approximately 1 cup each.

Cereals and breads: four servings of either 1 slice whole wheat bread or 1/2 to 3/4 cup whole grain cereal.

Meats, poultry, fish, beans: two servings of 2 to 3 ounces each.

Dairy products: 1 cup lowfat milk or 1 ounce cheddar cheese or 1/2 cup cottage cheese twice a day for adults; four times a day for teenagers; three times a day for younger children.

Drink plenty of water throughout the day—8 cups per day is recommended.

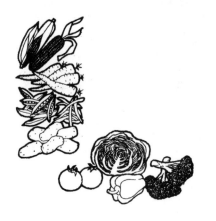

Sample daily menu

Breakfast:
- Cereal (oatmeal or other non-sugar) with 1/2 cup skim or low fat milk and a small amount of honey and/or fruit (once a week or so you may wish to have one or two eggs as an alternative).
- 1/2 cup fruit juice or 1/2 grapefruit.
- 1 slice whole wheat bread.
- Cup of coffee or, preferably, herbal tea.

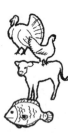

Lunch:
- Either a sandwich made with 2 slices of whole wheat bread or pita; fresh cooked turkey or tuna (packed in water); thin slice of cheese; lettuce, tomato, and or alfalfa sprouts; small amount of mayonnaise (preferably lite).
- Or a large salad made with any fresh vegetables you may have on hand, perhaps with tuna, chopped chicken or cottage cheese, and topped with a small amount of dressing. A slice of whole wheat bread or toast may go good with your salad.

Dinner:
- Dinner salad.
- Baked or broiled fish or poultry (skinless). Ground turkey is good in any dish where you might otherwise use hamburger.
- Steamed vegetables (fresh or frozen).
- Either a baked potato garnished with herb seasonings and a small amount of margarine, or herb seasoned rice or pasta.
- A cup of plain yogurt with fresh fruit for desert.
- You may wish to have a cup of herb tea or a small glass of wine with your meal.

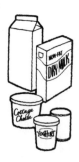

TABLE OF FOOD COMPOSITION

Item	Measure	Calories	Carbos.	Protein	Fat	Dietary Fiber
Beverages						
Beer, light	12 oz.	95	5.0	.9	.0	.0
Beer, regular	12 oz.	148	13.2	.9	.0	.0
86 proof liquor	1 oz	105	.0	.0	.0	.0
Wine, red	3.5 oz.	75	3.0	.2	.0	.0
Wine, white	3.5 oz.	80	3.0	.1	.0	.0
Coffee	1 cup	Tr	.5	Tr	.0	.0
Tea	1 cup	0	.1	.0	.0	.0
Cola drinks, reg.	12 oz.	160	40.0	.0	.0	.0
Fruit soft drinks	12 oz.	170	44.0	.0	.0	.0
Dairy Products						
Cheddar cheese	1 oz.	112	.4	7.0	9.4	.0
Mozzarella-part skim	1 oz.	80	1.0	8.0	5.0	.0
Parmesan	1 oz.	130	.8	12.0	9.0	.0
Cottage cheese-2%	1 cup	203	8.2	31.0	4.4	.0
Nonfat dried milk	3.2 oz.	325	47.0	32.0	.5	.0
Skim milk	1 cup	86	11.8	8.4	.4	.0
Lowfat milk-2%	1 cup	121	11.7	8.12	4.7	.0
Whole milk	1 cup	150	11.4	8.0	8.2	.0
Chocolate milk,whole	1 cup	208	25.8	7.9	8.5	.0
Plain Yogurt, whole	1 cup	139	10.6	7.9	7.4	.0
Plain yogurt, low-fat	1 cup	144	16.0	11.9	3.5	.0
Ice cream	1 cup	269	31.7	4.8	14.3	.0
Ice milk	1 cup	184	28.9	5.2	5.6	.0
Egg, raw	1 lg.	79	.6	6.1	5.5	.0
Egg white, raw	1 lg.	15	.3	3.6	1.0	.0
Egg yolk, raw	1 lg.	65	.1	2.8	5.6	.0
Desserts & Sweets						
Brownies,2X2X3/4"	1 pc.	146	15.3	2.0	9.4	1.0
Devils food cake, no icing,2X3X2"	1 pc.	165	23.4	2.2	7.7	.0
Chocolate icing	1/4 cup	359	46.3	2.2	9.6	.0
Chocolate milk bar	1 oz.	147	16.1	2.2	9.2	.0
Choc. chip cookie	2-1/2"dia.	51	6.0	.6	3.0	.0
Oatmeal cookie	3" dia.	63	10.3	.9	2.2	.0
Bran muffin	each	125	17.2	3.1	6.0	3.2
Glazed doughnut	each	235	24.0	4.0	13.0	.0
Honey	1 tbsp.	64	17.3	.1	.0	.0
Beet or cane sugar	1 tbsp.	46	11.9	.0	.0	.0
Jams & preserves	1 tbsp.	54	14.0	.1	.0	.0
Apple Pie,1/6 of 9"	1 pc.	410	61.0	3.4	17.8	.0
Pecan pie,1/6 of 9"	1 pc.	515	71.00	7.0	32.0	.0
Fruits, Nuts & Juices						
Apple, raw with peel	1 med.	81	21.0	.3	.0	4.5
Apple juice, unsw.	1 cup	117	29.5	.2	.0	.0
Avocado, fresh	1/2 med.	162	7.4	1.9	19.0	2.2
Banana, raw	1 avg.	105	27.0	1.2	.3	4.0
Cantaloupe	1/2 avg.	95	22.3	2.0	.7	2.7
Grapefruit	1/2 med.	41	10.8	.8	.1	1.1
Orange	1 avg.	64	16.0	1.3	.3	2.6
Orange juice, unsw.	1 cup	112	25.8	1.7	.5	.0
Peach	1 med.	35	10.0	1.0	Tr	2.3
Pear	1 med.	100	25.0	1.0	1.0	3.8
Pineapple	1 cup	77	19.0	1.0	1.0	1.8
Pineapple juice	1 cup	140	34.0	1.0	.3	.0
Raspberries	1/2 cup	30	14.2	1.1	Tr	4.6
Strawberries	1 cup	45	10.0	1.0	1.0	2.1
Watermelon, diced	1 cup	50	11.0	1.0	1.0	.0
Dates, pitted	10 med.	230	61.0	2.0	Tr	6.2
Raisins, packed	1/2 cup	239	64.0	2.1	.5	5.0
Almonds, raw	1/4 cup	212	6.9	6.6	19.5	5.1
Peanuts, roasted	1/4 cup	210	7.4	9.4	17.5	2.9
Peanut butter	1 tbsp.	95	3.2	5.0	8.1	1.2
Meat, Poultry & Seafood						
Chuck roast	4 oz.	226	.0	19.7	18.8	.0
Ground beef, lean	4 oz.	307	.0	28.0	21.3	.0
Ground beef, reg.	4 oz.	327	.0	26.7	24.1	.0
Turkey,chop'd,cooked	1 cup	240	.0	41.0	7.0	.0
Beef liver, fried	4 oz.	247	9.3	30.7	9.3	.0
Chicken breast	4 oz.	187	.0	36.0	4.0	.0
Chicken thigh	4 oz.	188	.0	30.0	5.0	.0
Turkey,roasted, dark	4 oz.	213	.0	32.0	8.0	.0
Turkey,roasted, white	4 oz.	180	.0	33.3	4.0	.0
Frankfurter	each	145	1.0	5.0	13.0	.0

Item	Measure	Calories	Carbos.	Protein	Fat	Dietary Fiber
Pork chop, broiled	3.1 oz.	275	.0	24.0	19.0	.0
Ham, cured	4 oz.	273	.0	24.0	18.7	.0
Bologna	2 slices	180	2.0	7.0	16.0	.0
Pork link, 1 oz ea.	1 link	50	Tr	3.0	4.0	.0
Bacon, reg.	3 pcs.	110	Tr	6.0	9.0	.0
Salami, cooked	2 slices	145	1.0	8.0	11.0	.0
Bass	4 oz.	118	.0	21.4	2.4	.0
Flounder or sole, baked, no margarine	4 oz.	107	Tr	22.7	1.3	.0
Halibut-broiled w/but	4 oz.	187	Tr	26.7	8.0	.0
Lobster	1 lb.	413	2.3	76.7	8.6	.0
Shrimp, fresh	4 oz.	103	1.7	20.5	.9	.0
Tuna, oil packed	4 oz.	220	.0	32.0	9.3	.0
Tuna, water packed	4 oz.	180	.0	40.0	1.3	.0
Dressings, Oils & Fat						
Mayonnaise	1 tbsp.	101	.3	.2	11.2	.0
Blue or roquefort	1 tbsp.	76	1.1	.7	7.8	.0
Italian, regular	1 tbsp.	83	1.0	.0	9.0	.0
Thousand island	1 tbsp.	60	2.5	.1	6.0	.0
Soy sauce	1 tbsp.	12	1.7	1.0	.2	.0
Butter	1 tbsp.	102	Tr	.1	11.5	.0
Margarine, regular	1 tbsp.	100	Tr	Tr	11.0	.0
Soft margarine	1 tbsp.	68	.0	.0	7.6	.0
Safflower oil	1 tbsp.	124	.0	.0	14.0	.0
Catsup	1 tbsp.	15	1.0	Tr	Tr	.0
Mustard	1 tbsp.	5	Tr	Tr	Tr	.0
Vegetables, Legumes, & Juices						
Alfalfa Sprouts	1 cup	10	1.0	1.0	.6	1.5
Asparagus, boiled	1 cup	45	8.0	5.0	1.0	1.5
Baked beans w/pork	1/2 cup	155	24.0	8.0	3.5	8.3
Kidney beans, dark	1/2 cup	115	21.0	7.5	.5	9.6
Green beans,steamed	1/2 cup	23	5.0	1.0	.0	2.0
Broccoli, cooked	1 cup	50	10.0	6.0	.5	5.6
Brussels sprouts	1 cup	65	13.0	6.5	.6	4.6
Cabbage, cooked	1 cup	29	6.2	1.6	.3	4.0
Carrots, froz.-cooked	1 cup	55	12.0	1.4	.3	4.6
Carrots, raw	1 med.	42	9.7	1.1	.2	2.5
Carrot juice	1 cup	96	22.2	2.5	.0	.0
Cauliflower,steamed	1 cup	28	6.0	2.9	.3	2.2
Celery, raw, diced	1 cup	20	4.7	1.1	.1	2.2
Corn, cooked	1 cup	137	31.0	5.3	1.7	7.8
Corn, cream style	1/2 cup	105	25.6	2.7	.75	3.0
Eggplant, cooked	1 cup	25	6.0	1.0	.4	5.0
Lentils, cooked	1/2 cup	106	38.6	15.6	Tr	3.7
Lettuce, iceberg	1 cup	5	2.2	.7	.1	1.4
Mushrooms, raw	1 cup	20	3.1	1.9	.2	1.8
Onions, cooked	1/2 cup	30	6.9	1.3	.1	1.6
Peas, steamed	1/2 cup	62	9.7	4.4	.3	5.0
Potatoes-baked w/skin	1 lg.	145	32.8	4.0	.2	3.9
French fries	10 pcs.	137	18.0	2.1	6.6	1.6
Potatoes, scalloped	1 cup	255	36.0	7.4	9.6	2.0
Spinach, steamed	1/2 cup	20	3.5	2.5	Tr	5.7
Squash, summer	1 cup	35	8.0	1.6	.2	4.0
Tomato, raw	1 med.	24	5.3	1.0	.3	1.8
Tomato juice	1 cup	46	10.4	2.2	.2	.0
Olives, green	4 med.	15	Tr	Tr	2.0	.0
Grains & Grain Products						
Bread, white enr.	1 slice	62	11.6	2.0	.8	.8
Bread, whole wheat	1 slice	56	11.0	2.4	.7	2.1
Pita, whole wheat	1 avg.	140	24.0	6.0	2.0	2.
Graham crackers	1 lg.	55	10.4	1.1	1.3	1.5
Saltine crackers	4 avg.	50	8.0	1.6	1.6	2.0
Noodles, egg enr.	1 cup	200	37.3	6.6	2.4	.0
Oatmeal, cooked	1 cup	145	25.2	6.0	2.4	5.7
Pancakes, plain enr.	4" dia.	62	9.2	1.9	1.9	1.5
Pancakes, whl. wheat	4" dia.	74	8.8	3.4	3.2	2.0
Pizza, cheese, 15"	1/8	290	39.0	15.0	9.0	.0
Popcorn, plain	1 cup	54	10.7	1.8	.7	2.0
Rice, white-cooked	1 cup	223	49.6	4.1	Tr	1.6
Rice, brown-cooked	1 cup	230	50.0	5.0	1.0	4.6
Shredded wheat bskt.	1 avg.	89	20.0	2.5	1.0	3.1
Bran Flakes, 40%	2/3 cup	101	24.9	1.5	.5	4.0
Corn Flakes	1 cup	110	24.4	2.3	Tr	2.8
Spaghetti, cooked	1 cup	190	39.0	7.0	.6	1.6

Recipes for Living Well

SUBSTITUTION TIPS

- Substitute 3/4 cup of honey for each cup of sugar that is called for in a recipe. In addition, for each cup of honey that is used, add 1/2 tsp. baking soda, and reduce the amount of liquid called for in the recipe by 1/4 cup. Bake at a slightly lower temperature.

- Use whole wheat pastry flour, cup for cup in place of white flour.

- Up to 1/3 of the flour called for in muffin, bread, pastry, cookie or cake recipes may be substituted with an equal amount of ground oat flour. Oat flour can also be used to thicken soups, stews and sauces. Seasoned oat flour makes a tasty coating for poultry and fish.

  To make ground oat flour, place 1 cup of uncooked oatmeal into the blender; cover and blend for about 1 minute, stopping occasionally to stir. Makes about 3/4 cup of oat flour.

- Ground turkey may be substituted for ground beef in most recipes, such as those for tacos, enchiladas, chili, spaghetti with meat sauce, sloppy Joes—even meatloaf and burgers. You may need to add a small amount of water to your pan when cooking, since the groundturkey contains very little fat.

ENTREES

LASAGNE

1 lb. Italian turkey sausage
1 garlic clove
1 Tbsp. whole basil
3/4 tsp. salt
1 (1 lb.) can tomatoes (2 c.)
2 (6 oz.) cans tomato paste (1-1/3c.)
10 oz. Lasagne, cooked
3 c. part skim ricotta or lowfat cottage cheese
1/2 c. grated Parmesan or Romano cheese
2 Tbsp. parsley flakes
2 beaten eggs
1 tsp. salt
1/2 tsp. pepper
1 lb. part-skim Mozzarella cheese, sliced very thin

Brown sausage slowly; spoon off excess fat, if any. Add next 5 ingredients. Simmer, uncovered, 30 minutes, stirring occasionally. Cook lasagne in large amount of boiling salted water until tender. Drain and rinse. Combine remaining ingredients, except Mozzarella cheese. Place half the noodles in 13 X 9 X 2" baking dish. Spread with half the cottage cheese filling. Add half of the Mozzarella cheese and half of the meat sauce. Repeat layers. Bake at 375° for about 30 minutes. Let stand 10 minutes before cutting in squares. Filling will set slightly. Makes 12 servings.

THYME SUMMER CHICKEN

4 skinless chicken breasts or skinless chicken parts if you prefer.
1/4 c. red wine vinegar
1 bay leaf, halved
2 tsp. onion powder
1 tsp. garlic powder
1 tsp. salt
1 tsp. thyme leaves, crushed
1/4 tsp. ground black pepper

In a small saucepan combine vinegar, water, bay leaf, onion and garlic powders, salt, thyme and pepper. Bring to a boil. Reduce heat and simmer, covered, for 2 minutes. Remove from heat; set aside to cool.

Pierce chicken with tines of fork, place in a tight-fitting container. Add cooled marinade; turn to coat. Cover and refrigerate at least 2 hours or overnight. Remove bay leaf. Preheat oven to 350°. Place chicken on a rack in a shallow baking pan, reserving marinade. Bake chicken, uncovered, basting frequently with marinade until the chicken is cooked through, 50-55 minutes.

To grill chicken, first bake it for 30 minutes, then place it on a rack over slow burning coals. Grill until cooked through, turning and basting often with marinade—about 30 minutes. Makes four servings.

CHICKEN FAJITAS (Fa-hee-tas)

1 lb. boneless, skinless chicken breast cut in bite size cubes
2 Tbsp. vegetable oil
2 Tbsp. lemon juice
1 tsp. garlic powder
1 tsp. seasoning salt
1/2 tsp. ground oregano
1/2 tsp. pepper
1/8 tsp. liquid smoke flavoring
1 c. each green pepper strips, thin onion wedges and thin tomato wedges
1/2 c. mild taco salsa
8 hot corn or flour tortillas

In a medium bowl, combine first eight ingredients. Cover and refrigerate 6 to 8 hours to marinate. In a 10 inch skillet, heat 3 Tbsp. oil over high heat until very hot. Saute half of meat until beginning to turn white—about 30 seconds Add half of green pepper and onion; continue cooking 1 to 2 minutes or until crisp-tender; remove all from skillet. Repeat with remaining chicken, pepper and onion—in additional oil, if needed. Return all of chicken, pepper and onion to skillet. Add tomato and 1/2 cup salsa; simmer for 1 minute longer while tossing chicken and vegetables. Serve immediately with additional salsa. Makes 4 servings. Serve with vegetarian refried beans and shredded lettuce.

OVEN BAKED MEXICAN CHICKEN

4 skinless, boneless chicken breasts
1 tsp. salt
1/3 c. whole wheat flour
1 tsp. chili powder
1/2 c. uncooked brown rice
2 tsp. chili powder
1 small onion, finely chopped
1 garlic clove , minced
1 green pepper, finely chopped
1 cup canned tomatoes, with juices

Mix salt, flour and chili powder. Roll each chicken breast in flour mixture. Place the chicken into a pyrex pan and bake in a 350° oven for 10 minutes. Then broil until browned—watch very closely.

In small mixing bowl, place brown rice, 2 tsp. chili powder, chopped onion, garlic, green pepper, and tomatoes; mix well. Pour mixture over the chicken breasts. Making sure the chicken is covered completely, bake in a 325° oven about 50 minutes or until the rice is cooked. Check after about 20 minutes to make sure there is enough liquid in the pan. Add water or chicken broth if too dry; however, there should not be too much liquid in pan, but rather a thick gravy or sauce. Makes 4 servings.

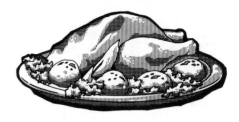

SWEET AND SOUR CHICKEN

1 lb. boneless, skinless chicken breasts, cut in cubes
2 Tbsp. oil
1 garlic clove, minced
1 c. green pepper strips
1 c. carrot strips
1-1/4 cups chicken broth or boullion
1/2 cup soy sauce
3 Tbsp. vinegar
3 Tbsp. honey
1/2 tsp. ginger
1 can chunk pineapple in juice (unsweetened)
1-1/2 c. quick brown rice

Saute chicken in oil until lightly browned. Add garlic and vegetables and stir fry for 2 to 3 minutes. Add boullion, soy sauce, vinegar, honey, ginger and pineapple with juice. Bring to a full boil. Stir in rice. Cover and cook until rice is tender. Makes 4 servings.

DEEP-DISH PIZZA

For thick crust, use two loaves of frozen whole wheat bread dough; for thin crust, use just one loaf. Thaw and press dough into a 15 X 11 X 2-1/2" pan; allow it to rise while you prepare other ingredients.

1 lb. turkey Italian sausage
1 lb. ground turkey
1 c. sliced mushrooms
3/4 c. chopped onions
1 c. chopped green pepper (optional)
1 qt. Italian sauce
1 lb. part skim Mozzarella cheese
1/2 c. Parmesan cheese

Cook sausage and ground turkey until browned. Add mushrooms, onions, green peppers and Italian sauce, and let simmer for 5 minutes. Pour mixture onto pizza crust; top with Mozzarella cheese; sprinkle with Parmesan cheese. Bake at 400° for 20-25 minutes or until crust is baked. Makes 12 servings.

SALMON-STUFFED MANICOTTI

12 large Manicotti
1/2 Tbsp. salt
3 qts. boiling water
1 can (15 oz.) salmon
1 c. lowfat cottage cheese
1 cup fresh or frozen chopped broccoli
1/2 tsp. grated lemon peel
Dash of nutmeg, salt, & pepper
3 Tbsp. margarine
3 Tbsp. whole wheat flour
2 vegetable bouillon cubes
2 c. boiling water
2 1/2 c. chopped fresh mushrooms
2 tsp. lemon juice

Gradually add Manicotti and salt to 3 qts. boiling water so that water continues to boil. Cook uncovered, stirring occasionally, until tender. Drain in colander.

While Manicotti are cooking, drain salmon and flake into medium bowl. Add cottage cheese, broccoli, lemon peel, nutmeg, salt and pepper. Stir lightly until just mixed. Fill each Manicotti with mixture; set aside.

In small saucepan, melt margarine. Stir in flour and cook over low heat, stirring constantly, until mixture thickens. Add bouillon cube to 2 cups water and stir until dissolved. Slowly add to flour mixture, then cook, stirring until mixture thickens. Add mushrooms and lemon juice and cook 2 - 3 minutes or until mushrooms are just tender. Pour all but 1 cup mushroom sauce in bottom of a 13" X 9" baking dish. Place stuffed pasta in dish and pour remaining sauce on top. Cover with foil. Bake at 375*, 25 - 30 minutes or until bubbly and hot.

Calories per serving approximately 266. Makes 6 - 8 servings.

LASAGNE-SALMON PINWHEELS

8 lasagne
1/2 Tbsp. salt
3 qts. water
1 can (15-1/2 oz.) salmon
1 container (15 oz.) part skim ricotta cheese
3 c. chopped fresh spinach (stems removed)
2 Tbsp. minced onion
2 Tbsp. grated Parmesan cheese
1-1/2 tsp. grated lemon peel
1/8 tsp. pepper
1 can (14-1/2 oz.) stewed tomatoes

Add lasagne and salt to rapidly boiling water, making sure the water continues to boil. Cook uncovered, stirring occasionally, until tender. Drain in colander.

While the lasagne is cooking, drain salmon and reserve liquid. Break salmon into small chunks in bowl; set aside. In another bowl, stir together ricotta cheese, spinach, onion, Parmesan cheese, lemon peel and pepper until blended. Add salmon chunks and toss gently.

Spread salmon mixture evenly over each lasagne leaving a 1/2 inch border at each end. Roll up and place pinwheel side up in greased 2-1/2 or 3 quart casserole dish. Stir salmon liquid into tomatoes. Spoon tomatoes around lasagne pinwheels. Cover and bake at 375° for about 30 minutes or until bubbly. Makes 8 servings, 274 calories each.

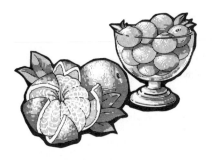

MISC. DISHES

QUICK FRUIT SHAKE

1/3 c. uncooked oatmeal
1 c. skim milk
4 ice cubes
1 Tbsp. honey
1/2 - 1 banana
1 peach, or any other fruit in season
1/4 tsp. vanilla

Place oatmeal in blender, cover and blend on high for 1 minute, stopping occasionally to stir. Add remaining ingredients and blend until smooth. Makes 2 cups.

COLE SLAW

1 head green cabbage (chopped)
1/2 Tbsp. salt
3/4 c. mild flavored honey
1/2 c. water
1/2 c. vinegar
1 tsp. mustard seed

Soak cabbage in 2 c. water and 1/2 Tbsp. salt for 1/2 hour. Pour off brine and add dressing made by mixing honey, water, vinegar, and mustard seed, mix. Add 3 cups chopped celery, and/or grated carrots, chopped red cabbage, or a small can of pimento, for color.

RICE PILAF

1/4 tsp. lemon juice
3 Tbsp. tomato paste
1/2 tsp. ground cinnamon
1/2 c. orange juice
1/2 tsp. grated orange rind
1/2 tsp. honey
Dash of salt and pepper (to taste)
2 c. chicken bouillon or broth
1 c. brown rice

Mix all ingredients, bring to boil, stir. Cover pot and simmer until nearly cooked (30 minutes). Let covered pot stand (off heat) for 10-15 minutes before serving. Serve alone or in a casserole with chicken. Makes about 4 cups.

PANCAKE & WAFFLE MIX

4 c. whole wheat pastry flour
1 c. soy flour
2 Tbsp. baking powder
1 Tbsp. salt
1/2 c. non-fat milk powder or 2/3 c. instant

Stir dry ingredients together and store in tightly covered jar. Makes about 6-1/2 cups of mix.

For pancakes or waffles:

1-1/2 c. mix
1 or 2 eggs
2 Tbsp. oil
2 Tbsp. honey

Enough water to make a thick batter for pancakes or a thin batter for waffles.

For extra fluffy pancakes, separate the eggs; whip the whites until stiff; fold into the batter. For variety, add chopped apples and cinnamon or any fruit or berries that may be in season.

STRAWBERRY SHORTCAKE

2 eggs (beaten)
1/2 c. honey
1 tsp. vanilla
4 Tbsp. hot water
1 c. whole wheat pastry flour
1 tsp. baking powder
1/4 tsp. baking soda
1/4 tsp. salt

Beat eggs. First add honey, then add vanilla and water; mix. Add last four ingredients; mix. Pour into greased and floured 8 X 8" pan. Bake at 350° for 35-40 minutes. Cut into 9 pieces.

1 pt. fresh strawberries, hulled and cut in quarters
3 Tbsp. honey
Enough water to cover.

Mix and chill in refrigerator for at least 2 hours, for flavors to blend. Serve over shortcake.

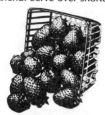

PEANUT BUTTER BALLS

1-1/3 c. freshly ground peanut butter
2/3 c. honey
1-1/2 c. dry milk powder
1/2 c. wheat germ
1-1/2 tsp. coconut flavoring

Mix thoroughly. Refrigerate dough about 1 hour in a covered container. Roll into small balls.

FRENCH APPLE PIE

6 c. sliced tart apples
1-1/4 tsp. ground cinnamon
1/4 tsp. ground nutmeg
3/4 c. skim milk
2 Tbsp. margarine, softened
2 eggs
3/4 c. honey
1/2 c. whole wheat baking mix
Streusel (directions below)

Grease 1-1/2 x 10" pie pan. Mix apples and spices; turn into pie pan. Beat remaining ingredients, except streusel, until smooth—about 1 minute with beater. Pour over apples in pie pan. Sprinkle with streusel. Bake until knife inserted comes out clean—55-65 minutes.

Streusel: Mix 1 c. whole wheat baking mix, 1/2 c. chopped nuts, 1/2 c. packed brown sugar and 3 Tbsp. firm margarine until crumbly.

BRAN MUFFINS

1 c. whole wheat pastry flour
1 c. bran
2 tsp. baking powder
1/4 tsp. baking soda
1/4 c. oil
1 egg
1/4 c. honey
1-1/2 c. skim milk or 1-1/2 c. buttermilk
1 c. raisins

Combine dry ingredients and raisins in a bowl. Combine wet ingredients, and then add to dry ingredients. Stir briefly. Spoon into muffin tins with liners. Bake at 400° for 17 minutes. Makes 12 muffins.

WHOLE WHEAT PIE CRUST

1 c. whole wheat pastry flour
1/4 tsp. salt
1/4 c. vegetable oil
3 Tbsp. ice water

Preheat oven to 375°. Put flour and salt in 9 inch pie pan and mix well. Measure the oil in a large measuring cup. Add the ice water to the oil and mix well, using a fork. Slowly add the liquid to the flour mixture in the pie pan, mixing it with the same fork. Continue mixing until all ingredients are well blended.

Press into shape with your fingers, making sure that the crust covers the entire inner surface of the pie pan evenly. Prick the bottom of the crust with a fork in several places and place in a 375° oven for 20-25 minutes, or until golden brown if the recipe calls for a prebaked pie crust.

ZUCCINI NUT BREAD

3 eggs
3/4 c. oil
1-1/2 c. honey
2 c. shredded zuccini
2 c. whole wheat pastry flour
1/4 tsp. baking powder
2-3/4 tsp. baking soda
1 tsp. salt
3 tsp. cinnamon
2 tsp. vanilla
1 cup coarsely chopped walnuts

Beat eggs. Add honey, oil and zuccini; mix well. Add dry ingredients; mix. Add vanilla & nuts. Pour into two loaf pans (5 X 9") that have been oiled & floured. Bake at 350° for 1 hour, or until toothpick inserted comes out clean.

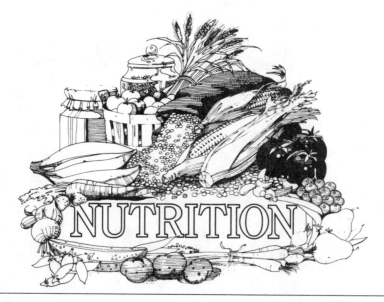

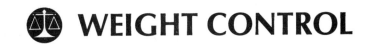

Since the turn of the century, the average American has gained an average of 22 pounds. With all the marvelous checks and balances that are naturally built into the body, you might reasonably wonder why weight control requires so much special effort on the part of so many people.

Here are some of the reasons for this rapid rise:
• fats in the American diet have increased by 40 percent;
• starches (which tend not to produce fat) have decreased by 43 percent;
• many highly processed foods—few of which even existed in 1900—have become staples;
• greasy fast foods have gained great popularity.

At the same time, hard work is now far more likely to consist of pushing a pencil than pushing a plow; going on a round of errands usually means driving the car rather than riding a horse or taking a hike; and the popular notion of recreation has shifted from enjoying a pleasant walk to viewing the latest episode of a favorite TV show.

These truly momentous changes in the way we live have occurred far too rapidly for our bodies to fully adjust as biological systems.

How Much Weight Is Right For You?

Not surprisingly, proper weight is very much an individual matter. For example, a six foot football player might have a proper weight of 230 pounds, while a sprinter of the same age, sex and height might have a proper weight of 165 pounds. That's because what matters is not actually your weight, but the amount of fat you're carrying as compared to your productive body mass—your muscle, bone and organ tissue. In this country, as many as eight out of ten people carry more fat than is desired for optimal efficiency.

For the average person, a healthy ratio of body fat to total body mass ranges from 15 to 19 percent for adult males, and from 18 to 22 percent for females. An ideal percentage of body fat for a well conditioned male athlete is 8 to 15 percent; for a female athlete, 12 to 18 percent.

Use these formulas to estimate your ideal weight:

Adult male: Allow 106 pounds for the first five feet of height, and add 6 pounds for each additional inch (plus or minus adjustment for frame).

Adult female: Allow 100 pounds for the first five feet of height, and add 5 pounds for each additional inch (plus or minus adjustment for frame).

Adjustment for frame: Subtract 10% from the result for a light frame; add 10% for a heavy frame (see the note in the lower part of the margin at right).

Maintaining a weight that is right for you is an important aspect of preserving your health for a lifetime. If you are of normal weight for a person your height, sex and body build, you are likely to live longer, have more energy and feel better than if your weight is above normal. In addition, overweight is associated with many health problems, including atherosclerosis, heart disease, stroke, cancer, kidney problems, diabetes, high blood pressure, malnutrition, low energy level, inactivity and impaired self-image. It's clearly worth the effort to keep your weight under control.

Of course, for most people the question isn't whether or not it's worth the effort. What it usually boils down to is how to do it—reliably, safely and relatively painlessly so you can go on living as you like without losing your capacities along the way.

Body composition. The proportion of your total body mass that is properly composed of fat depends upon your sex, body build and patterns of activity. Generally speaking, a healthful body composition for women is about 18 percent, and for men about 13 percent.

A few people, like male marathon runners, may get to as low as 5 percent; while Eskimo peoples, who live active lives in close contact with the antarctic elements, may be in excellent physical condition yet carry a higher than average percentage of body fat as protective insulation.

What Is Your Ideal Weight?

The average person can approximate his or her ideal weight from this chart:

Ideal Weights for Various Frame (Bone) Sizes					
Your	**Female**			**Male**		
Height	**Small**	**Med**	**Large**	**Small**	**Med**	**Large**
5'0"	90	100	110	95	106	117
5'1"	95	105	115	101	111	123
5'2"	100	110	122	106	118	130
5'3"	104	115	126	112	124	136
5'4"	108	120	132	117	130	143
5'5"	113	125	137	122	136	150
5'6"	117	130	143	128	142	156
5'7"	122	135	148	133	148	163
5'8"	126	140	154	139	154	169
5'9"	131	145	159	144	160	176
5'10"	135	150	165	149	166	183
5'11"	140	155	170	155	172	189
6'0"	144	160	176	160	178	196
6'1"	149	165	181	166	184	202
6'2"	153	170	187	171	190	209
6'3"	158	175	192	176	196	216
6'4"	162	180	198	182	202	220

*To determine your frame size, measure the distance around the wrist of your dominant hand (the one you write with):

	Female	Male
Small frame	under 6"	under 6-1/2"
Medium frame	6 to 6-1/2"	6-1/2 to 7"
Large frame	over 6-1/2"	over 7"

Surplus fuel is stored in special fat cells located throughout your body. Every pound of excess fat requires an extra 200 miles of capillaries, taxing your entire cardio-respiratory system for its support.

One pound of fat represents 3,500 calories of potential energy.

Since one hour of brisk walking burns roughly 350 calories, 10 hours of walking—with no increase in food consumption—will eliminate about one pound of fat. This means that taking a one hour walk (at a rate of 4 miles per hour) each day for a year will allow you to shed approximately 36 pounds of fat.

How Many Calories Are Enough?

You can estimate the approximate number of calories you need to maintain your present weight from this table (you need less if you intend to lose weight):

Calories Per Day At Various Activity Levels						
Ideal	**Under Age 40**			**Over Age 40**		
Wght	**Low**	**Med**	**High**	**Low**	**Med**	**High**
90 lb	1350	1530	1800	1170	1440	1800
100	1500	1700	2000	1300	1600	2000
110	1650	1870	2200	1430	1760	2200
120	1800	2040	2400	1560	1920	2400
130	1950	2210	2600	1690	2080	2600
140	2100	2380	2800	1820	2240	2800
150	2250	2550	3000	1950	2400	3000
160	2400	2720	3200	2080	2560	3200
170	2550	2890	3400	2210	2720	3400
180	2700	3306	3600	2340	2880	3600
190	2850	3230	3800	2470	3040	3800
200	3000	3400	4000	2600	3200	4000

Low activity means sedentary work, without regular exercise.

Medium activity means sedentary work with moderate regular exercise (jogging 3 miles/day).

High activity means either physically strenuous daily work or exercising to a level that burns 500 calories per day (e.g., jogging 5 miles daily).

Adopt a Long-Term Strategy for Success

The first principle of an effective weight control program is to make sure that it is capable of working over the long haul. Crash weight loss programs are notorious for their failure rates because they are almost always nutritionally unsound to begin with. Any weight that is lost, and often much of this is water, tends to be quickly regained when the temporary program is discontinued and the old patterns are resumed. Effective weight control is an important strategic element of your general lifestyle, rather than a "quick-fix" reaction to your present condition.

Another weak strategy is the use of large amounts of protein—often taken as a food substitute—for the purpose of losing weight. Unless conducted under close professional supervision, and with the administration of carefully formulated nutritional supplements, such programs are ineffectual at best, and they can be quite dangerous.

Weight change = nutritional input - energy output in the form of activity

Your body forms fat when the food you eat contains more calories, or energy value, than you are able to use at the time. On the other hand, when you expend more calories than you're taking in, some of your body fat is burned to make up the difference, thereby reducing your overall body weight. So you can lose weight by eating properly, by becoming more active, and, of course, by doing both at the same time.

How Many Calories Do You Need?

If you are under age 40, you very likely expend an average of about 12 calories per pound of ideal body weight each day to maintain normal body temperature and to fuel basic body processes. If you are over 40, this requirement changes to about 10 calories per pound of ideal weight per day. Beyond that, you probably need a few hundred additional calories to supply the energy needed for earning a living and conducting your other affairs (more if your work involves heavy labor). So, for example, if your ideal weight is 150 pounds and you're under 40, that's roughly 2,000 total calories per day. Although a few individuals seem to become overweight while consuming even fewer calories, most need about these amounts—derived from whole unprocessed foods—to maintain lean, energetic bodies.

What Is The Role of Genetics

The rate at which fat cells multipy and accumulate at various points throughout your body is related to your heredity. This means that if you take in excess calories, you are likely to store the resultant fat as your parents did. However, if you don't take in those excess calories, you won't develop the surplus fat cells either. Persons with a genetic predisposition to obesity more readily produce fat when they consume surplus calories, and they more easily retain fat once it has been produced.

Nutritional Input

Food bulk is not what produces fat. Surplus calories produce fat. By increasing your intake of fiber-rich fruits, vegetables, whole grains and legumes, while decreasing your intake of high calorie meats, sugars, fats and alcoholic beverages, you will have gone a long way toward gaining control of your weight. Ounce for ounce, carbohydrates contain only half the calories of fat, so replacing fats, fried foods and fatty meats with unrefined carbohydrates cuts your caloric intake considerably, without giving you the feeling that you're starving yourself in the process.

As a matter of fact, your efforts at weight control can actually be frustrated by depriving your body of the regular food intake to which it has grown accustomed. Your body may react to a lack of food by conserving as much fat as possible, apparently as a protection against prolonged deprivation. For this reason, skipping meals and engaging in starvation diets are ineffective as weight control strategies.

How Many Calories Are You Consuming?

One effective step that you can take to help gain control of your weight is to determine the approximate number of calories you are taking in on the average. The best way to do this is by keeping a record of everything you eat, while tallying up the total calories consumed each day. Since most people are not willing to carry on a detailed count of their calories over an extended period, a periodic sampling of perhaps 5 to 7 days in duration can probably give you a fair idea of just how many calories you're taking in, and where they are coming from. A form is provided on page 68 for keeping an Eating Diary.

Activity

In addition to proper nutritional intake, weight control is a matter of energy expenditure—that is, burning up calories through physical activity. When you are generally inactive, your body chemistry is altered so that fewer calories are burned as you perform all your normal daily activities. On the other hand, when you regularly engage in physical activity of some intensity, your muscles produce more of the chemicals that convert blood sugar and fat into energy. You're also signalling to your body that it needs strength and endurance to meet the demands you're placing upon it, so more protein is diverted to the building of muscle and organ tissue. These changes persist in your body long after the period of activity itself, so that even while you are sitting at your desk or sleeping in bed, your body is burning more calories and preparing itself for the next exertion. This yields dividends in the form of more muscle and bone, less fat, more energy and improved concentration.

Think Thin

Understanding the process by which fat is produced is only part of the solution. To gain lasting weight reduction requires altering any patterns of thought, feeling or behavior that may be contributing to your weight problem. If you have been overweight for some time, it's likely that you have adjusted your self image so that you now think of yourself as "being fat"—at least to some extent. And, when you think of yourself in this way, it's entirely consistent for you to feel and act as a "fat person" might.

One of the most important steps you can take—perhaps the easiest step—is to readjust your self image so that you think of yourself as a thin, trim, healthy and active person. Initially this is done through the use of your imagination. By seeing, feeling and accepting yourself as one who is naturally well-proportioned, you prepare the way for acting toward the realization of this result.

Feel Trim

Your feelings or emotions are also a part of your behavioral patterning. Eating is sometimes used in an effort to satisfy other needs, such as the need for love, social acceptance or excitement. Or it may be used to relieve uncomfortable feelings like loneliness, boredom, tension, fear or depression. These feelings may then become associated with excessive or otherwise nutritionally unbalanced eating, often bringing effects which are exactly the opposite of those intended—more depression, more loneliness, or whatever.

Digestion is aided by the churning action of the stomach; an action which is most efficient when the stomach is not over-filled. If you are overweight, your stomach muscles may be stretched and out of tone. By not filling your stomach, you give it an opportunity to recover its normal healthy shape and tone, while permitting the most efficient digestive action to take place.

To help assure that you do not overfill your stomach, eat slowly, and finish eating before your stomach feels full. Remember that the more food you habitually eat, the more it will take to give you the sensation of fullness.

In referring to the Table of Food Composition, use these guidelines to estimate the number of calories contained in various foods,

- For unprocessed carbohydrates and protein, multiply the number of grams of food by 4 to arrive at the approximate number of calories.
- For fats, multiply grams of food by 9.

This clearly illustrates the high calorie density of fats as compared to other foods.

For example:, a cup of low-fat (2%) cottage cheese carries these numbers of calories for its various components:

Carbos: 8.2 grams x 4 cal/gm = 32.8 cal

Protein: 31.0 grams x 4 cal/gm =124.0 cal

Fat: 4.4 grams x9 cal/gm = 39.6 cal

Total calories 196.4 cal

> *The key factor in weight control is balancing the calories you're taking in with the calories you're expending in your daily activities.*

Some Weight Loss Tips

If you have some extra fat to lose, take advantage of any obvious opportunities you have for reducing your caloric intake. For example:

Put less food on your plate.

Stop eating **before** you feel full.

Leave some food on your plate.

Don't go back for seconds.

Remove your plate when you have finished.

Leave leftovers for another meal.

Pass up desserts, or have fresh fruit instead.

Stay active—get daily exercise.

Don't starve yourself (go without food).

Don't rely upon diet pills.

Avoid greasy fast foods.

Shop for groceries when you're full.

Don't eat while doing other things.

Avoid snacks between meals.

Remember to eat vegetables.

Avoid double applications of fats—butter and salad dressing or sour cream and cheese.

Care for yourself.

Avoid soft drinks and fruit "flavored" drinks.

Control alcohol intake, which relaxes both self-discipline and appetite control.

Become aware of any self-defeating associations that may exist between your patterns of eating and your emotional state. Then identify things you can do which can be more realistically expected to resolve the difficulty. When you notice that you are experiencing the emotion, bring your thin self image to mind, and take whatever action you have determined to be more effective.

To develop a clear image of yourself as a thin person, remember another time when you may have been more trim. If you have any pictures of yourself as a thin person, get them out and look at them. Visualize yourself now as you were then. Allow yourself to feel what you felt like at that time. You may want to put a picture up where you can see it each day. If you have always been overweight, then find models for the way you want to look in magazines. When you see someone whose shape you admire, visualize yourself as having that shape. On the other hand, never allow yourself to make unfavorable comparisons between yourself and anyone else, as this will tend to undo the good work you have done on your new self image.

Act Trim

If you're overweight, set realistic goals for yourself, bearing in mind the length of time it took to gain the extra weight in the first place. Be patient...shedding a pound or two each week is plenty. Over a year that adds up to between 50 and 100 pounds!

Keep Track of Your Progress

The Weight Control Progress Chart on page 66 will help you to keep track of your weight. Use the Living Well Daily Performance Record to keep an eye on how you're doing with these five key wellness factors which relate most directly to weight control:

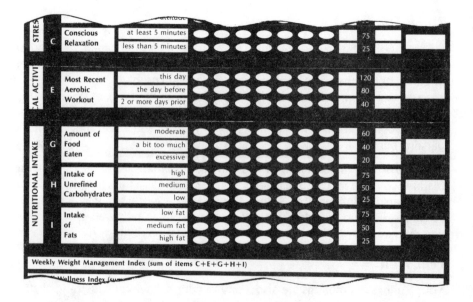

At the bottom of the Daily Performance Record is a place for tallying up your weekly scores for these five items which are specifically related to weight control. This total will allow you to see at a glance just how well your behavior is supporting the achievement of your weight control objective.

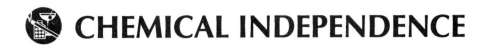

A dependency may arise from the regular use of any drug taken for the purpose of altering your mood. The drugs most commonly used for mood alteration are tobacco, caffeine, alcohol and sedatives, amphetamines, cocaine, marijuana, narcotics and hallucinogens.

Each of these substances has physical effects in addition to its psychoactive, or mind-altering properties. Most of them can seriously damage your body when taken in large amounts or over an extended period of time.

With repeated use, the body may also develop a tolerance for the drug, requiring larger or more frequent doses for the same mood-altering effect. With certain drugs, such as barbiturates, for example, a tolerance for the mood-altering effects develops more rapidly than does tolerance for the physical effects. In this case, as users take more and more of the drug to obtain the same "high," they unwittingly approach the threshold of toxic, or even lethal, overdose.

In addition to the dangers associated with the drugs themselves, the way in which they are taken may introduce another set of risks. Three ways are most common: oral ingestion, inhalation, and injection. Depending upon the toxicity of the substance, oral ingestion places the mouth, throat and digestive system at risk. Inhalation places the mouth, throat and lungs, or in some cases the delicate nasal and sinus membranes, at risk. Injection heightens the risk of overdose, and introduces the possibility of needle contamination and vascular damage. Because of the very real risk of contracting AIDS (Acquired Immune Deficiency Syndrome) by this means, use of shared or non-sterile needles must now be viewed as an imminently life-threatening practice.

Dealing with chemical dependency

Addictions to alcohol, barbiturates, cocaine, heroin and other substances are now recognized as severe illnesses which manifest themselves both physically and behaviorally. In most areas, qualified professional assistance is readily available to treat these illnesses during their acute stages, and to provide valuable follow-through services.

It's important to bear in mind that denial is a central characteristic of chemical abuse problems. Denial is a serious obstacle which is faced not only by the abuser himself, but also by others who are affected. Before the recovery process can begin, this pattern of denial must be broken. If you suspect that a friend, associate, family member, or you yourself may have a drug abuse problem, seek out and take advantage of the best available professional assistance.

Among the alternatives are self-help groups—such as Alcoholics Anonymous—which have assisted untold numbers of people in similar circumstances. To get started you may want to use a telephone help-line. 1-800-COCAINE is available nationally, and you may find a local help-line within the government listings in your phone book.

Avoiding potential dependencies

If you would like to cut down on your use of alcohol, or discontinue your use of tobacco or any other chemical substance, the discussion which follows is for you. In the example, smoking is used to illustrate the procedures, but the same approach can be applied to the elimination of any potential dependency.

Step 1. Clearly determine for yourself that you are entitled to live your life independent of any potentially damaging chemical substances; that you are

Physical and Psychological Dependence

Regular use of any mood altering substance produces at least some degree of psychological dependence—that is, a reliance upon it to make you feel good. Certain of the substances also produce a physical dependence because of adjustments the body makes to accommodate them. After these adjustments have been made, the body becomes distressed when it is deprived of the drug. The most physically addictive substances are barbiturates, alcohol, cocaine, narcotics and tobacco. Others which appear to be physically addictive, though to a lesser extent, are amphetamines, caffeine and marijuana.

INCREASED RISK OF DYING OF VARIOUS DISEASES DUE TO SMOKING:

Disease Category	Increase in Risk (%)
Coronary heart disease	70 - 300
Emphysema and other chronic airway obstructions (excluding asthma)	1000 - 2000
Lung cancer	700 - 1500
Laryngeal cancer	500 - 1300
Oral cancer	300 - 1500
Esophageal cancer	400 - 500
Bladder cancer	100 - 300
Pancreatic cancer	100
Kidney cancer	50
Peptic ulcer disease	100

A person who smokes one pack of cigarettes or less per day would be assuming risks at the lower end of the spectrum. Those smoking more than a pack a day would assume risks at the higher end. Most important, **the *smoker* assumes all these risks at the same time.**

(Source: American Council on Science and Health)

What is heavy drinking?

The Institute on Alcohol Abuse defines light drinking as under four drinks per week, moderate drinking as four to 14 drinks, and heavy drinking as over 14 per week. By this definition, one drink equals 1-1/4 ounces of whiskey, 5-ounces of wine, or 12-ounces of beer. So if you average more than two such drinks per day, then you're a heavy drinker.

How do you know if someone is drinking too much?

If you wonder about it, the person probably is, whether the person is you or someone else. If alcohol has become an important part of any person's emotional or physical needs, a problem is present. If you see that problem, don't ignore it.

entirely capable of granting yourself this independence; and that you are unwilling to settle for anything less than enjoying the full measure of physical health, emotional balance and psychological freedom that is your birthright.

It is in the nature of dependencies that they present the illusion of holding power over the will of the individual. If you're like most people, you aren't entirely comfortable with the idea that anything has power over your will to act in your own best interests. Yet many people are reluctant to challenge an ingrained habit for fear that there may be a high price to pay in terms of physical discomfort and mental distraction. In short, they are held hostage by the threat of losing the temporary sense of well-being which they have become accustomed to giving themselves through the use of the chemical. Eventually their inherent capacity for the experience of joy itself may be compromised by the gradual transfer of this great personal power from themselves to an external object—a chemical substance.

If you have grown accustomed to using one or more chemical substances—tobacco, alcohol, caffeine or other drugs—take the first step now. Consciously claim your right to stay well and to live free of any encumbering dependencies. For now, do this without concern for how you will accomplish it, and without anticipating any difficulty or discomfort. Simply establish this as a necessary principle for healthful, joyous living, which somehow or other you are determined to implement within your life.

Step 2. Closely observe and record your use of any chemical substance that has the potential of becoming a dependency. Observe without exercising judgment and without attempting to intervene at this point. Notice as many details as possible—the circumstances, associates, environment, your feelings and thought patterns, your moods, your words and your behavior. And remember, do nothing but watch and keep a record at this time . . . without even a judgment. Simply pay close attention to all the dynamics of your use of the substance as an interested, yet completely detached observer. Give no thought to the idea of altering your patterns, other than to keep a record of your usage (see form on page 70), including the amount, the time, the circumstances, the effects—both immediate and subsequent—and any other observations you may make. If you find that you're resisting this step, simply take note of that fact, along with everything else, and continue to observe and record whatever is taking place.

Step 3. To the extent possible, rearrange your environment so that you can avoid any triggers that you've identified. Plan activities which can substitute for those which occasion your use of the substance. If drinking a cup of coffee after breakfast is closely associated with smoking a cigarette, change to another drink, or drink at another time.

Step 4. Practice the other Living Well techniques, especially conscious relaxation and aerobic exercise.

Step 5. Adopt the point of view that you are freeing yourself of any dependency that may be a threat to you. What you are setting out to accomplish is the feat of becoming, with the totality of yourself, a person who is truly a non-smoker, a non-drinker, a non-drug user or whatever.

To approach smoking cessation as a smoker who is trying to quit is virtually guaranteed to engage you in a knock-down, drag-out fight with yourself. While continuing to see yourself as one who smokes—a smoker, you're demanding of yourself the elimination of the very behavior that goes along with being a smoker—smoking. Instead of engaging in this type of internal conflict, adopt the strategy of actually becoming a non-smoker. In this way you can live out the thoughts, feelings and behaviors that flow naturally from the enjoyment of this essential state of well-being.

You can accomplish this through the determined use of your creative imagination during your goal clarification exercises. As you know, the more comprehensive and realistic the image of yourself as a non-smoker becomes, the easier it is for you to live it out in your daily life. The experience of millions of people has shown that it is entirely possible to reprogram yourself as a non-smoker who never again feels inclined to touch a cigarette.

Along with developing a new self-image, give yourself a few instructions for handling the situations that are likely to come up. For example, when you awaken in the morning, be prepared to carry on as a non-smoker—that is, without giving the matter any attention—until something comes up which raises the issue of smoking. If a friend who thinks of you as a smoker offers you a cigarette, or if something else occurs which brings up the question as to whether or not you would like to smoke, be prepared to immediately ask yourself one simple question: "Am I a smoker; or am I a non-smoker?" Do this before you have had an opportunity to think of anything else, or to engage in any deliberations that might otherwise be triggered by the offer of a cigarette.

If the answer you receive is that you are a smoker, then you know that your reprogramming activity is not complete. If the answer is that you are a non-smoker, then simply act accordingly—the situation calls for no further attention or thought.

When someone asks you if you have quit smoking, acknowledge that you no longer smoke, without allowing yourself to become involved in anyone else's idea of how difficult it is to "quit." Until you have accumulated some time as a non-smoker, it may be best not to discuss what you are doing unless you are talking with someone who can assist you. Without even thinking about it yourself, simply allow yourself to be the person you have chosen to become.

On the other hand, if you should discover that you are still a smoker, then return once again to the creative process of goal clarification, with the patient determination that you are, in fact, becoming a non-smoker, non-drinker etc., and that it is simply a matter of time until this result is fully realized in your life. Avoid negative self-judgments. For example, don't allow yourself to turn a slip into a sweeping generalization about your ability to deal with the habit—an over-reaction which is likely to precipitate a full relapse into the undesired behavior.

Of course, you may supplement your private efforts with professional assistance if that appears to be warranted.

Maintain A Watchful Eye

The Living Well Daily Performance Record (page 60) reviews these factors:

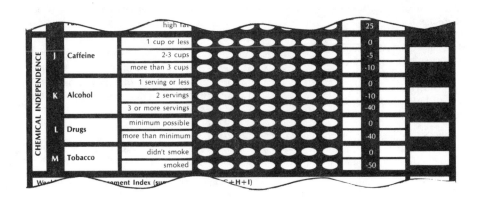

Amphetamine is the drug most commonly used in sports today, despite the well-documented fact that it does not improve performance. One reason for its continued use is that it unrealistically inflates subjective perception of performance. Among the risks: heatstroke is often associated with the use of amphetamines—it can be lethal in combination with hot weather and strenuous competition. It also impairs judgment, decreases split-second problem-solving ability, increases the risk of injury by masking fatigue, and drastically extends recovery time following an athletic event.

Alcohol

Misuse of alcohol is a factor in about 200,000 deaths a year. It is associated with half of all traffic deaths, many of them involving teenagers. Given that about two thirds of all adults drink at least occasionally, it is perhaps not surprising that ten million are estimated to be alcoholics or problem drinkers.

Like the sedatives, alcohol is a drug which depresses the central nervous system. In small doses, alcohol has a tranquilizing effect on most people, though it appears to stimulate a few. It first acts on those parts of the brain which affect self-control and other learned behaviors, giving rise to unusual aggressiveness in some people. Even one or two drinks can significantly impair a driver's judgment and reaction time. In large doses, alcohol can dull sensation while impairing muscular coordination, memory and judgment. Repeated drinking of alcohol produces tolerance and can lead to strong physical and psychological dependence, accompanied by severe withdrawal symptoms.

When taken in quantity over an extended period of time, alcohol can damage the liver, heart and brain. Cirrhosis, one of the ten leading causes of death, is largely attributable to alcohol. Alcohol use is also associated with cancers of the liver, esophagus and mouth. While even moderate drinking is a risk during pregnancy, excessive drinking may lead to severe infant abnormalities. On average, heavy drinking reduces life span by about 10 years.

In a culture where alcohol is commonly used as a social lubricant, the probability of repeated exposure to alcohol is high. While for the majority of people, light consumption of alcohol appears to be relatively safe, for many others this is very definitely not the case. The ingestion of alcohol is ill-advised during pregnancy, in combination with certain medications, or when recovering from some illnesses.

Alcohol, even in small quantities, is also unsafe for a large and diverse population of people who seem to possess a physical predisposition to alcohol addiction. That is, when they engage in the practice of drinking, they're more likely than others to drink to excess, and to eventually fall prey to a dependency. Some people are exceptionally sensitive to the mood altering effects of alcohol, while some others have a higher than average tolerance for these effects. Those in the latter category may experience less intense mood-altering effects when drinking moderate amounts of alcohol, yet beyond a certain threshold point, they become just as intoxicated as anyone else who has consumed a like amount. These biologically predetermined all-or-nothing setups carry with them a higher susceptibility to the formation of a chemical dependency.

Unfortunately, there is no reliable way of testing for such predispositions beforehand. Conse-quently millions of people discover the problem only after they have already fallen prey to it.

Amphetamine

(Speed, Crank, Crystal)

Amphetamine is a stimulant often referred to as an "upper." At this time, some 2.2 million Americans use the drug in the misguided belief that it is beneficial for overcoming fatigue and losing weight.

During the 1940's, 50's and 60's amphetamines (including dextroamphetamine and methamphetamine) were hailed as new wonder drugs, enabling users to go for extended periods without food or rest. Their use steadily grew as the drugs were widely prescribed for problems such as depression, lethargy, and fatigue. Eventually, however, it was their ability to suppress appetite, coupled with America's obsession with thinness, that led to their tremendous growth in popularity during the 60's and early 70's, when they gained widespread use as diet pills.

Gradually, serious health hazards were linked to amphetamines. At the same time, evidence was mounting regarding their ability to produce a high degree of tolerance, and to establish a powerful psychological dependence. During the late 70's, awareness of the dangers associated with them brought a rapid decline in their medical use, and along with it their pharmaceutical availability. Nevertheless, amphetamines and their lookalikes have remained available on the street for those who would use them. Continued use of these drugs, despite the obvious risks, may be attributable to the very powerful rush of ex-hilaration which is initially experienced.

Methamphetamine, also known as "crystal," is the most potent form of the drug. As a powder, it can be injected, inhaled or taken orally. It is also available as a pharmaceutical tablet under the tradename Desoxyn. During a "run" involving extended use, feelings of fatigue and hunger may be so effectively blocked that users grossly overexert themselves, failing to take food or rest for days—perhaps even weeks—at a time. Such episodes tax the system intolerably, producing rapid deterioration of physical and psychological well-being. Among the possible effects: vitamin and mineral deficiencies; lowered resistance to disease; damage to the lungs, liver and kidneys; fatigue, anxiety, insomnia, depression; and the onset of delusional states or even full-blown toxic psychosis.

The effects of ingested amphetamines, or "crank," are virtually identical to those produced by crystal, though at similar dosage levels they are somewhat less intense.

Lookalikes are tablets and capsules which simulate prescription amphetamines, and which usually consist of blends of caffeine, ephedrine, and phenylpropanolamine—compounds that can be found in a number of over-the-counter stimulants, diet pills, decongestants and antihistamines. Despite the fact that their ingredients are sold legally, lookalikes are not safe, and have been implicated in a number of deaths, mostly due to massive sudden increases in blood pressure, resulting in cerebral hemorrhage.

Anabolic Steroids

These hormonal supplements are taken by many athletes with the goals of accelerating body-building and improving performance. While in some cases they may temporarily support the accomplishment of these goals, they also exact an extremely high price for the short-term gains which they provide. When the administration of steroids is discontinued, the extra body bulk which they induced quickly dissipates, though their damaging side effects may not. They are usually taken either orally or by injection, often with needles shared among a number of young athletes.

Because of their strong associations with self-image and their temporary effect, discontinuing their use is extremely difficult for many people.

Known side effects include acne, alteration of sexual desire, sterility, dizziness, fainting, headache, lethargy, irritability, a tendency toward aggressive behavior and violence, premature balding, elevation of serum cholesterol, increased risk of heart attack at an early age, ulcers in the intestinal tract, liver disease, cancer and possibly a long-term effect on the brain, with irreversible personality changes.

Caffeine

Caffeine, which stimulates the central nervous system, can produce anxiety, gastritis, heartburn and sleeplessness.

Cocaine

In 1986 an estimated 22 million Americans sampled cocaine, and at least 5 million use it regularly. While cocaine was once thought to be non-addictive, it is now known to be perhaps the mos ddictive drug of all, and one of the hardest drug habits to shake.

Chemically, it performs dual functions: it is both a powerful stimulant, and an anesthetic that numbs whatever tissue it touches. It produces feelings of alertness and energy that peak quickly and then rapidly fade. Users often feel confident and in control. It also blocks appetite and erases fatigue, giving it the appearance of a performance booster.

Cocaine can be inhaled, injected (intravenously, subcutaneously or intramuscularly), or smoked. It comes in various forms, including a white crystalline powder that is inhaled or injected; in purified forms such as free base and crack; and in the form of a crude coca paste which may be smoked on tobacco cigarettes. When inhaled or injected, the "high" lasts from 30 minutes to an hour; when smoked, it lasts from 3 to 5 minutes. The risk of fatal overdose is increased with smokable forms of cocaine because it is difficult to estimate dosage. After the initial euphoria has passed, a severe "crash" is often experienced, which may last for as long as a week.

The adverse physical effects of cocaine use include irregular heart beat, hypertension, elevated body temperature, dizziness, severe headache, impotence, liver damage, constriction and possible rupture of the coronary arteries, epileptic seizures, paralysis, strokes, coma, and sudden death. Many of these effects, including the most serious, can occur even among first time users. Inhaling cocaine vapors may cause lung damage, including chronic congestion, coughing and pain in the lungs and throat. Extensive cocaine use burns out the body, producing malnutrition and weight loss, and may permanently scramble intra-brain communications.

On the psychological side, suspiciousness, anxiety, irritability and insomnia are among the early symptoms of cocaine dependence. Symptoms of longer term dependence include bizarre behavior, severe agitation, hallucinations, extreme paranoia, depression and suicidal desperation.

Depressants (Sedatives)

The primary effect produced by all depressant drugs is suppression of activity within the central nervous system. In general, these drugs slow down all of the bodily and mental functions. While low doses usually produce a feeling of relaxation, not dissimilar to the effects associated with social drinking of alcohol, high doses may produce drowsiness, loss of muscle coordination, lethargy, disorientation, low blood pressure, confusion, memory impairment, rage reactions, personality alterations, and symptoms resembling drunkenness. Three different types of depressant drugs are reviewed here: barbiturates, benzodiazepines and methaqualone.

Barbiturates

Barbiturates, including compounds such as amobarbital (Amytal), pentobarbital (Nembutal), secobarbital (Seconal), butabarbital (Butisol) and phenobarbital, are among the most prescribed psychoactive drugs in the United States. They are most often used medically as mild tranquilizers or sleeping pills.

Barbiturates are misused by at least one million Americans, and an estimated 30,000 are addicted to them. Regular use over a period of time can induce psychological and physical dependence as well as a very rapid build-up of tolerance to the euphoric effects. Eventually the amount needed to obtain the euphoric effects may exceed a lethal dose, without the user knowing it, thus making barbiturates a leading cause of drug

overdose fatalities. Combinations of barbiturates with other depressants, particularly alcohol, are extremely risky. Barbiturates are often used to "come down" after a prolonged period of amphetamine use. They are also used as a substitute drug by heroin addicts. Barbiturates taken during pregnancy may cause addiction within the newborn child, as well as increasing the risk of birth defects.

Barbiturate withdrawal is often more severe than heroin withdrawal, with abrupt withdrawal sometimes leading to convulsions which may produce permanent disability or even death. For this reason it is essential that withdrawal from barbiturate addiction be professionally supervised.

Benzodiazepines (Valium)

Benzodiazepines are a group of sedatives, or tranquilizers, including such trade names as Valium, Tranxene, Librium, Ativan, and Serax. Approximately 9 percent of the population over 14 years of age has used tranquilizers, and close to 5 percent use them regularly. These non-barbiturate sedative-hypnotic drugs have been widely used medically to treat anxiety, tension and insomnia, initially with the belief that they were non-addictive substitutes for the highly addictive barbiturates.

It is now known that regular use of these sedatives can develop a tolerance, so that increasingly larger doses are needed to produce the same effects. Furthermore, frequent use over a prolonged period of time, can produce a physical dependence involving severe withdrawal symptoms. More commonly, however, a psychological dependence develops, particularly in those who use these drugs to cope with routine daily stress.

Methaqualone (Quaaludes)

Another group of more powerful tranquilizers, based upon the generic compound methaqualone, includes such products as Optimil, Sopor, Somnifac, Mequin and Quaalude.

Because for some time these were alleged to be "safe," non-addicting sedatives, they gained wide usage among individuals seeking relief from the anxieties of daily living. However, they are now known to have potent dependence-producing properties, with a high potential for abuse and overdose. Withdrawal carries approximately the same risk as withdrawal from barbiturates, and can be quite severe in the case of a major addiction. Alcohol, barbiturates and other anti-anxiety compounds can intensify the drug's effects and increase the risk of overdose.

Intoxication with methaqualone is similar to intoxication with barbiturates or alcohol and subjects the individual to similar risks—that is, accidents due to confusion and impaired motor coordination, and death by overdose. Beyond its initial euphoric effects, methaqualone has been known to induce headaches, hangover, fatigue,

dizziness, drowsiness, torpor, menstrual disturbance, dry mouth, nosebleeds, diarrhea, skin eruptions, lack of appetite, numbness, and pain in the extremities. More severe cases of overdose can result in restlessness, muscle spasms, convulsions, delirium, coma and death.

Hallucinogens

Hallucinogens include LSD, mescaline, psilocybin and a range of other chemicals with names such as DMT, STP, and MDA. Hallucinogens are capable of altering time and space perception; changing feelings of self awareness and emotion; changing one's sense of body image; increasing sensitivity to textures, shapes, sounds and taste; bringing on visions of luminescence, flashes of light, kaleidoscopic patterns and landscapes. They can also induce hallucinations, and feelings of religious experience.

Hallucinogens are not known for producing either physical or psychological dependence, although tolerance quickly develops in the use of some. Some psychological dependence has been observed in long-term LSD users, but has rarely been reported as a consequence of other hallucinogenic use. Cross tolerance is also common, so that an individual who has recently taken LSD will generally show a reduced response to mescaline and psilocybin, for example.

Flashbacks—recurrence of hallucinogenic experiences—have been reported over periods ranging from a few months to more than a year after last LSD use. At high doses, MDA, which has an amphetamine base, has occasionally been implicated in serious physical reactions requiring medical treatment.

Marijuana

Marijuana is currently used by an estimated 16 million persons. Over time, smoking five marijuana cigarettes a week is as damaging to the lungs as smoking about six packs of cigarettes a week. Marijuana use affects hormonal balance, including both sex and growth hormones. It may reduce fertility in women and sperm count in men. Marijuana may be especially harmful during adolescence—a period of rapid physical and sexual development. Marijuana may also have a toxic effect on embryos and fetuses. THC, the main psychoactive ingredient in marijuana, is measurable in urine up to ten weeks after usage, and even longer in blood samples. This means that frequent usage has a cumulative effect—increasingly destablilizing the body chemistry. This may be reflected in loss of sex drive, exaggerated mood swings and a general feeling of lethargy. Many of these effects appear to quickly recede after usage is discontinued.

Narcotics
(Heroin, Opium, Morphine, Codeine)

Narcotics generally refer to drugs derived from the oriental poppy plant, as well as to some synthetic compounds that have morphine-like effects, such as meperidine (Demerol) and methadone. These drugs are produced in the form of tablets, capsules, powders and liquids. They may be ingested, inhaled (sniffed), or taken intravenously.

Opiate narcotics can rapidly produce substantial psychological and physical dependence, with the degree of physical dependence determined by the quantity, frequency and duration of use. For frequent users and higher dosage levels, tolerance develop quickly. Withdrawal effects after heavy chronic use are severe and painful, resembling those associated with alcohol and barbiturate withdrawal.

There are between 400,000 and 750,000 heroin addicts in the United States. Methadone, which is used in the management of opiate narcotic dependence, often produces a dependency of its own, and hence is also widely abused. Heroin is usually taken intravenously, whereas methadone is more commonly, though not always, taken by mouth—in tablet or liquid form.

The effects of a typical intravenous dose of heroin may last from two to six hours or more, while those of methadone may last many times longer. The effects include an initial surge of pleasure, then a prolonged period of dropping in and out of a drowsy, dream-like state, accompanied by a feeling of contentment and detachment.

Immediate responses to the drug also frequently include such effects as reduced breathing and heart activity, heaviness in the arms and legs, dizziness, constriction of the pupils and reduction of visual acuity, drowsiness, lethargy, loss of concentration, apathy, itching, skin rash, dry mouth, warming of the skin, increased perspiration, constipation, suppression of hunger, lowered sex drive, nausea and sometimes vomiting. As doses get higher these effects become more acute, sometimes resulting in insensibility and unconsciousness. Very high doses may initiate coma, shock, respiratory arrest and even death.

PCP

(Phencyclidine)

This drug is a white crystalline powder, soluble in water, and is most commonly smoked or ingested. The majority of users are aged 12 to 18. Street names include "angel dust," or simply "dust," as well as "super weed," "THC" or "Tic" because it is sometimes misrepresented as synthetic marijuana. While it does not appear to be physically addictive, with prolonged use a very strong psychological dependence can be developed.

Physiological symptoms include increases in heart rate and blood pressure, sweating, salivation, and flushing of the skin. Low doses produce auditory, visual, time and other sensory distortions, the most consistent of which is deadening of sensation in the extremities and loss of muscle control. It may interfere with hormones which relate to normal growth and development in the adolescent user. Depending upon the individual, the range of generalized reactions can vary from complete immobility to hyperactivity or even violence. Because it produces a loss of feeling, injuries involving cuts, bruises and torn muscles or ligaments often occur with higher doses. Common psychological effects include paranoia, severe agitation, social withdrawal, feelings of isolation, and bizarre delusions. Its use impairs concentration, learning performance and social adjustment. Adverse effects may persist for many months after use has been discontinued.

Tobacco

Cigarette smoking is considered by many authorities to be the largest single preventable cause of illness and premature death in this country. Tobacco is associated with an estimated 320,000 premature deaths a year, and another 10 million people currently suffer from debilitating chronic diseases caused by smoking. Disease and lost productivity due to smoking are estimated to cost the economy of the United States about $65 billion a year—more than $2 for every pack of cigarettes consumed.

The use of tobacco quickly forms a powerful psychological dependence and tolerance. It is associated with premature aging of the skin; gum disease; stomach ulcers; gangrene of the extremities; heart and blood vessel diseases; stroke; chronic bronchitis and emphysema; cancers of the mouth, throat, lung, pancreas, bladder, cervix and stomach.

Smoking during pregnancy tends to retard fetal growth while raising the risk of miscarriage, prematurity, stillbirth, death during the first day of life and sudden infant death syndrome (SIDS). Children of smoking parents, especially infants, are more likely to suffer respiratory ailments, chronic ear infections and stunted growth. Spouses of smokers have a 30 percent increased risk of developing lung cancer.

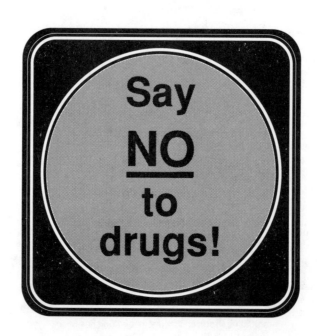

In addition to the various Living Well factors already discussed, there are a number of measures that you can easily take to further reduce your risk of serious illness and injury.

Drive safely:
- Make certain that you and your fellow travelers have fastened your seatbelts.
- Maintain your vehicle in good working order—especially such important safety items as lights, windshield wipers, brakes and tires.
- Observe the speed limit and other traffic rules.
- Never allow yourself or someone you know to operate a motor vehicle after drinking too much.

Physical examinations:
- Keep an eye on your blood pressure. The higher number (systolic) should be about 120, and the lower number (diastolic) about 80—shown as 120/80. High blood pressure, or hypertension, increases the risk of heart and arterial disease by as much as 800%. You can reduce your blood pressure by controlling your weight, moderating salt intake, engaging in regular exercise, and lowering the level of cholesterol in your bloodstream.
- Have yourself checked for cancer. Tobacco and nutrition are the primary behavioral factors influencing the development of cancer. For those who do not smoke, up to 70% of the total cancer risk is related to patterns of nutritional intake.
- Periodically check the levels of cholesterol and high density lipoprotein (HDL) in your blood. A recommended frequency for this check is once each year.

Cholesterol, which is essential to normal functioning, is a waxy, fatty substance that occurs in blood and body tissue. Too much cholesterol greatly increases the risk of developing heart and arterial disease in the form of atherosclerosis, or hardening of the arteries.

HDLs, on the other hand, serve as an important antidote to the potential clogging effects of cholesterol in the bloodstream. By coating the inside of the artery walls with a protective layer of grease, they help to prevent the build-up of fatty deposits. And they act as a scrubbing agent by dissolving those fatty deposits which do occur.

The ratio of total cholesterol to HDL in the bloodstream is perhaps more significant than simply the level of cholesterol alone. For men, the ratio should be less than 5, and preferably less than 4.5 (for example, if total cholesterol is 180, then HDLs should be at least 36, and preferably 40 or above). For women, the ratio should be still lower: no higher than 4, and preferably 3.5 or less (women naturally tend to have more HDLs than men).

Environmental pollutants:
- In the home, exercise proper precautions in the storage and use of all toxic substances.
- As much as possible, avoid passive smoking. Living or working with people who are smoking significantly increases risk for smoking-related illnesses. In the case of pregnant women, living with a smoker produces 66% as severe an effect on birthweight as if the mother herself were smoking.
- In your community, do what you can to help retard the pollution of natural resources, and to restore the natural beauty and life-supporting quality of the environment.

The three major risk factors for heart disease are:
- High blood cholesterol
- High blood pressure
- Cigarette smoking

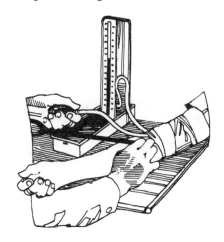

Cholesterol in the blood

Maintaining a proper level of cholesterol in your bloodstream is an important factor in protecting against heart and arterial disease:

Blood cholesterol level (mg/dl)	Risk of heart disease
180 or less	Safe level
180 to 200	+25% risk
200 to 220	+100% risk
220 to 240	+150% risk
240 to 260	+200% risk
260 to 300	+300% risk
above 300	+400% risk

The American Institute for Cancer Research offers these guidelines for lowering cancer risk:

- Reduce the intake of dietary fat from the current average of approximately 40% to a level of 30% of total calories.
- Increase the consumption of fruits, vegetables and whole grain cereals.
- Consume salt-cured, smoked and charcoal-broiled foods only in moderation.
- Drink alcoholic beverages only in moderation.

What is your present risk of cancer?

This simple self-test was designed by the American Cancer Society to help you assess your risk of certain common types of cancer. Please bear in mind that these are not the only known risk factors, and that the point values provide only a general indication of your risk with respect to the factors mentioned.

Directions

In the space provided, mark the number of points (shown in parentheses) that corresponds to your answer.

COLON-RECTUM CANCER (Males & Females)

WHAT IS YOUR AGE
- under 50 (1)
- 50 to 59 (3)
- 60 or over (12)   _____

HAS ANYONE IN YOUR IMMEDIATE FAMILY EVER HAD:
- colon cancer (5)
- one or more polyps of the colon (2)
- neither (1)   _____

HAVE YOU EVER HAD:
- colon cancer (12)
- polyps of the colon (5)
- ulcerative colitis (4)
- none of these (1)   _____

HAVE YOU EXPERIENCED BLEEDING FROM THE RECTUM
(other than from hemorrhoids or piles)
- yes (10)
- no (1)   _____

TOTAL [ ]

Score

- **under 10:** You have a low risk for colon-rectum cancer.
- **10 to 25:** You are at moderate risk—ask your physician whether you should be tested further.
- **over 25:** You are at high risk for this type of cancer. Consult with your physician regarding the frequency with which you should be tested.

Comments

With early detection, 80 percent of all bowel cancers can be cured. These cancers grow slowly, and they can be detected by means of examinations which your doctor can provide: a digital rectal exam, stool blood test, and proctoscopic exam.

SMOKING/LUNG CANCER (Males & Females)

YOUR AGE
- under 40 (1)
- 40-49 (2)
- 50-59 (5)
- 60+ (7)   _____

NUMBER OF CIGARETTES SMOKED PER DAY
- none (1)
- 1-9 (5)
- 10-19 (9)
- 20-39 (15)
- 40 or more (20)   _____

TYPE OF CIGARETTE*
- high tar/nicotine (10)
- medium tar/nicotine (9)
- low tar/nicotine (7)   _____

DURATION OF SMOKING
- under 15 years (3)
- 15 to 24 years (6)
- 25 or more years (12)   _____

TOTAL [ ]

*High T/N .... 20 mg. or more tar/1.3 mg. or more nicotine
Medium T/N .... 16-19 mg. tar/1.1-1.2 mg. nicotine
Low T/N .... 15 mg. or less tar/1.0 mg or less nicotine

Score

- **under 10:** As a non-smoker, you have a low risk for lung cancer.
- **10-25:** As a smoker, your risk of lung cancer is considerably increased.
- **over 25:** As a heavy cigarette smoker, your chances of getting lung and upper respiratory tract cancer are greatly increased. Consult with your physician if you develop a nagging cough, hoarseness, a sore or persistent pain in your mouth or throat.

Comments

Smoking causes 75 percent of lung cancers and 25 percent of all forms of cancer. The longer and heavier one smokes, the greater the risk. As soon as smoking is discontinued, the body starts to repair itself, and the risk of lung cancer gradually approaches that of non-smokers.

There is no safe cigarette. While smokers of low tar/low nicotine cigarettes do have a slightly lower lung cancer rate, their substantially elevated coronary heart disease rate is the same as that of high tar/nicotine smokers.

YOUR AGE
- under 40 (1)
- 40-49 (3)
- 50+ (6)   _____

YOUR ETHNIC GROUP
- Hispanic (1)
- Oriental (2)
- Black (2)
- White (3)   _____

YOUR FAMILY HEALTH HISTORY
- no breast cancer in immediate family (1)
- mother, sister, aunt or grandmother has
  had breast cancer (3)   _____

YOUR HEALTH HISTORY
- no breast cancer (1)
- previous breast cancer (3) _____

YOUR HISTORY OF PREGNANCIES
- first live birth before age 18 (1)
- first live birth at age 18-34 (2)
- first live birth at age 35 or older (4)
- no live births (3)   _____

TOTAL [   ]

Scores

- **under 5:** You have a relatively low risk for breast cancer. Perform monthly breast self-examinations, and have your breasts examined by your physician during check-ups.
- **5 to 10:** Your risk is somewhat elevated. In addition to monthly self-examinations and regular check-ups, periodic breast x-rays may be recommended by your physician.
- **10+:** Your heightened risk for breast cancer suggests that more frequent examinations and breast x-rays may be called for. Consult with your physician to discuss the appropriate frequency.

Comments

Breast cancer, the second leading cause of death in women, is almost 90 percent curable when detected early. Once the cancer has spread, however, the rate of cure drops to less than 50 percent. To safeguard against this form of cancer, all women over the age of 20 should do a monthly breast self-exam. Women between the ages of 20 and 40 also should have a doctor examine their breasts every three years. After the age of 40 women should have an examination annually and a mammogram, or breast x-ray, every one to two years. Women over 50 should have an annual mammogram.

HOW CANCER WORKS

Normally, the cells that make up the body reproduce themselves in an orderly manner so that worn-out tissues are replaced, injuries are repaired and healthy body growth proceeds.

Occasionally, certain cells undergo an abnormal change, triggering a process of uncontrolled growth. These cells may grow into masses of tissue called tumors—some benign and others malignant, or cancerous.

The danger of cancer is that it invades and destroys normal tissue. At the outset, cancer cells usually remain at their original site, and the cancer is said to be localized. Later, some cancer cells may invade neighboring organs or tissue. This occurs either by direct extension of growth or by becoming detached and carried through the lymph or blood systems to other parts of the body. The spread may be regional—that is, confined to one region of the body—as when cells are trapped by lymph nodes. If left untreated, however, the cancer is likely to eventually spread throughout the body, usually resulting in death.

Because cancer becomes more serious with each successive stage, early detection is important.

Most cancer cases in the United States are believed to be associated in some way to the physical surroundings and/or personal lifestyle. About 30% of all cancers are directly related to the use of tobacco, either alone or in conjunction with excessive consumption of alcohol.

Aside from not smoking, proper nutritional intake is the next most important factor in reducing cancer risk.

Exposure to toxic chemicals is another risk, though it is much less substantial than smoking and diet for most people who are not involved in high risk occupations.

CANCER'S SEVEN WARNING SIGNALS

1. Change in bowel or bladder habits
2. A sore that does not heal
3. Unusual bleeding or discharge
4. Thickening or lump in breast or elsewhere.
5. Indigestion or difficulty in swallowing
6. Obvious change in a wart or mole
7. Nagging cough or hoarseness

Consult with your physician if you should observe the occurance of any of these conditions.

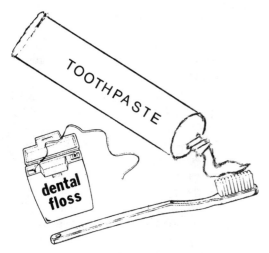

Dental hygiene

Your teeth are essential tools. They not only perform the basic digestive functions of biting and chewing food, but they also serve as an important feature of your countenance—especially your smile. When kept in good condition through a few simple maintenance techniques, they can be expected to last you for a lifetime with minimal difficulties. On the other hand, when they are not properly taken care of on a regular basis, there are a number of very troublesome problems which can arise, including bad breath, cavities, receding gums, gum disease, and gradual loss of teeth. The proper measures for care of your teeth include:

• Brush your teeth at least once each day, following the procedure recommended by your dentist.
• Floss your teeth daily. This prevents the buildup of bacterial in the crevices between your teeth, and is both important not only for the prevention of tooth decay, but also for avoiding the development of unpleasant mouth odor.
• Visit your dentist every six months for a checkup and cleaning.

AIDS:

Acquired Immune Deficiency Syndrome, (AIDS) is a deadly communicable virus for which there is no known cure at this time. An estimated 1.5 million Americans are presently infected with the AIDS virus, and are assumed to be capable of transmitting it. People may carry the virus indefinitely without manifesting symptoms.

Although the virus has been found in saliva and tears, it is thought to be transmitted only through contact with infected blood, semen or vaginal secretions.

Roughly 25% of AIDS cases are linked to the practice of sharing needles among intravenous drug users. The virus is transferred via minute traces of blood left on the needle or in the syringe.

70% of all AIDS cases to date are attributed to sexual transmission. Since it is assumed that one sexual contact with an infected person is sufficient to contract the virus, the risk of infection increases with each new sexual partner. The risk increases dramatically when the partner has engaged in sex with a number of different people during the past several years. The best protections against the sexual transmission of AIDS are abstinence and the careful use of condoms.

There is no evidence to indicate that the AIDS virus is transmitted by casual contact. Even relatives who have shared food and such items as towels with AIDS victims over an extended period of time have not been shown to contract the virus by these means.

Blood transfusions are now safe, but those received before March 1985, carried a slight risk (about 1 in 100,000) of involving contaminated blood.

Women infected with the AIDS virus can pass it on to their unborn children. About 1 in 3 babies of infected women have been infected; most have died.

There are no known cases of AIDS transmission by insects.

The Living Well program provides you with an efficient and enjoyable means of systematically building all these positive patterns of living into your accustomed way of life.

You'll note that, for the most part, Living Well focuses your attention on adding desirable new behaviors to your present way of life, rather than on changing or eliminating old behaviors. This new complex of healthful activities has the welcome effect of gradually easing out many of the less desirable patterns, often without raising even the hint of a struggle.

Live out your plan of action for the next six weeks. Make that commitment to yourself at the outset. Approach it as a six week experiment in taking charge of your life. Don't be bothered by any initial resistances you may feel—just accept them as a matter of course, and keep right on going.

If you have a personal goal for reducing your weight or resting heart rate, record your status at the beginning of each week in the progress charts provided for this purpose. You'll be able to keep track of your progress in all areas by recording your daily activity using the convenient Daily Performance Record. Then, at the end of each week, tally up your scores for the week, and enter them on your Long-Term Progress Record (if you wish, you can translate them into separate colors for a more dramatic visual effect).

Upon completion of each six-week cycle, you'll once again be ready to retake the Lifestyle Inventory. This provides you with a comprehensive picture of how you're doing with respect to the full array of wellness-related lifestyle factors, and prepares the way for you to establish new wellness goals for the next cycle.

Over the long term, you'll find that persistence and determination are your most valuable assets for Living Well. When you're not entirely satisfied with your progress, simply reaffirm your determination and continue to persist in the healthful course that you have chosen for yourself. Reinforce your new self-image—your personal wellness goal—every day with at least a few minutes of quiet, relaxed visualization, perhaps while driving your car or before dropping off to sleep at night. Then renew it again when you awaken in the morning. Do this until you become so familiar with this new image of yourself that any other ideas feel foreign to you. Don't allow yourself to indulge in any contrary visions of who you are, and who you are becoming. When they do occur, simply substitute your new self-image in their place.

And remember to reward yourself for your accomplishments. The changes you're making have great long-term value, and immediate rewards recognize and reinforce your success right now.

Always bear in mind that your life is entirely yours to live, and that you deserve the best, regardless of anything you may have experienced up to now. At first you may feel a little like you're swimming upstream—you and everyone else who knows you expect you to think, feel and act according to your familiar patterns. But soon you'll notice that you're becoming more comfortable acting in ways that are consistent with your new self-concept, and that your old patterns are beginning to feel like last decade's wardrobe—a little out of fashion. Let them go! Before you know it, you'll be completing your first six-week cycle, and you'll be successfully launched on a new, healthier way of living—***choosing your way to lasting health and well-being.***

So get yourself started right now—today. There's no better way for you to invest your time and attention. The payoffs are enormous, and they'll keep right on coming in, day after day, year after year for the rest of your life.

The Living Well program provides you with these 13 wellness-related objectives from which you may select your current set of personal wellness goals:

In the area of Stress Management:
- Conscious relaxation*
- Goal clarity and personal organization
- Attitude control

In the area of Physical Activity:
- Full-body stretching
- Cardio-respiratory activity*
- Body toning

In the area of Nutrition:
- Eating Independence*
- Unrefined carbohydrate intake*
- Fat intake*

In the area of Chemical Independence:
- Caffeine intake
- Alcohol intake
- Drug intake
- Tobacco use

*Weight management is accomplished through practicing these five of the thirteen Living Well objectives.

How to use the Daily Performance and Long-Term Progress Records

Keep a daily record of how well you're doing by filling in the appropriate dot for each Living Well objective.

Summarize your results at the end of each week:

1. First, count the number of dots you've filled in on each line; enter the totals in the "#" column.

2. Next, multiply these totals by the number given in the "X" column, and enter this product in the "=" column.

3. Add up the two or three products associated with each objective, and enter the results in the "Total" column.

4. Use these totals to arrive at your Weekly Weight Management and Living Well Indices.

5. Transfer all of your Weekly totals to the Long-Term Progress Record provided on page 67.

		OBJECTIVE		S	M	T	W	T	F	S	#	X	=	TOTAL
STRESS MANAGEMENT	A	Clarity and Personal Organization	clear & organized	○	○	○	○	○	○	○	☐	45	☐	☐
			a bit disorganized	○	○	○	○	○	○	○		30		
			poorly organized	○	○	○	○	○	○	○		15		
	B	Attitude Control	positive attitude	○	○	○	○	○	○	○	☐	90	☐	☐
			mostly positive	○	○	○	○	○	○	○		60		
			negative attitude	○	○	○	○	○	○	○		30		
	C	Conscious Relaxation	at least 5 minutes	○	○	○	○	○	○	○	☐	75	☐	☐
			less than 5 minutes	○	○	○	○	○	○	○		25		
PHYSICAL ACTIVITY	D	Full- Body Stretching	stretched	○	○	○	○	○	○	○	☐	60	☐	☐
			didn't stretch	○	○	○	○	○	○	○		20		
	E	Most Recent Aerobic Workout	this day	○	○	○	○	○	○	○	☐	120	☐	☐
			the day before	○	○	○	○	○	○	○		80		
			2 or more days prior	○	○	○	○	○	○	○		40		
	F	Most Recent Body Toning Workout	this day	○	○	○	○	○	○	○	☐	30	☐	☐
			1 or 2 days before	○	○	○	○	○	○	○		20		
			3 or more days prior	○	○	○	○	○	○	○		10		
NUTRITIONAL INTAKE	G	Amount of Food Eaten	moderate	○	○	○	○	○	○	○	☐	60	☐	☐
			a bit too much	○	○	○	○	○	○	○		40		
			excessive	○	○	○	○	○	○	○		20		
	H	Intake of Unrefined Carbohydrates	high	○	○	○	○	○	○	○	☐	75	☐	☐
			medium	○	○	○	○	○	○	○		50		
			low	○	○	○	○	○	○	○		25		
	I	Intake of Fats	low fat	○	○	○	○	○	○	○	☐	75	☐	☐
			medium fat	○	○	○	○	○	○	○		50		
			high fat	○	○	○	○	○	○	○		25		
CHEMICAL INDEPENDENCE	J	Caffeine	1 cup or less	○	○	○	○	○	○	○	☐	0	☐	☐
			2-3 cups	○	○	○	○	○	○	○		-5		
			more than 3 cups	○	○	○	○	○	○	○		-10		
	K	Alcohol	1 serving or less	○	○	○	○	○	○	○	☐	0	☐	☐
			2 servings	○	○	○	○	○	○	○		-10		
			3 or more servings	○	○	○	○	○	○	○		-40		
	L	Drugs	minimum possible	○	○	○	○	○	○	○	☐	0	☐	☐
			more than minimum	○	○	○	○	○	○	○		-40		
	M	Tobacco	didn't smoke	○	○	○	○	○	○	○	☐	0	☐	☐
			smoked	○	○	○	○	○	○	○		-50		

Weekly Weight Management Index (sum of items C+E+G+H+I)	☐
Overall Wellness Index (sums of all items)	☐

Keep a daily record of your performance by filling in the appropriate ovals–see margin of previous page for instructions.

DAILY PERFORMANCE RECORD – WEEK 2

		OBJECTIVE		S	M	T	W	T	F	S	#	X	=	TOTAL
STRESS MANAGEMENT	A	Clarity and Personal Organization	clear & organized	○	○	○	○	○	○	○	☐	45	☐	☐
			a bit disorganized	○	○	○	○	○	○	○	☐	30	☐	
			poorly organized	○	○	○	○	○	○	○	☐	15	☐	
	B	Attitude Control	positive attitude	○	○	○	○	○	○	○	☐	90	☐	☐
			mostly positive	○	○	○	○	○	○	○	☐	60	☐	
			negative attitude	○	○	○	○	○	○	○	☐	30	☐	
	C	Conscious Relaxation	at least 5 minutes	○	○	○	○	○	○	○	☐	75	☐	☐
			less than 5 minutes	○	○	○	○	○	○	○	☐	25	☐	
PHYSICAL ACTIVITY	D	Full-Body Stretching	stretched	○	○	○	○	○	○	○	☐	60	☐	☐
			didn't stretch	○	○	○	○	○	○	○	☐	20	☐	
	E	Most Recent Aerobic Workout	this day	○	○	○	○	○	○	○	☐	120	☐	☐
			the day before	○	○	○	○	○	○	○	☐	80	☐	
			2 or more days prior	○	○	○	○	○	○	○	☐	40	☐	
	F	Most Recent Body Toning Workout	this day	○	○	○	○	○	○	○	☐	30	☐	☐
			1 or 2 days before	○	○	○	○	○	○	○	☐	20	☐	
			3 or more days prior	○	○	○	○	○	○	○	☐	10	☐	
NUTRITIONAL INTAKE	G	Amount of Food Eaten	moderate	○	○	○	○	○	○	○	☐	60	☐	☐
			a bit too much	○	○	○	○	○	○	○	☐	40	☐	
			excessive	○	○	○	○	○	○	○	☐	20	☐	
	H	Intake of Unrefined Carbohydrates	high	○	○	○	○	○	○	○	☐	75	☐	☐
			medium	○	○	○	○	○	○	○	☐	50	☐	
			low	○	○	○	○	○	○	○	☐	25	☐	
	I	Intake of Fats	low fat	○	○	○	○	○	○	○	☐	75	☐	☐
			medium fat	○	○	○	○	○	○	○	☐	50	☐	
			high fat	○	○	○	○	○	○	○	☐	25	☐	
CHEMICAL INDEPENDENCE	J	Caffeine	1 cup or less	○	○	○	○	○	○	○	☐	0	☐	☐
			2-3 cups	○	○	○	○	○	○	○	☐	-5	☐	
			more than 3 cups	○	○	○	○	○	○	○	☐	-10	☐	
	K	Alcohol	1 serving or less	○	○	○	○	○	○	○	☐	0	☐	☐
			2 servings	○	○	○	○	○	○	○	☐	-10	☐	
			3 or more servings	○	○	○	○	○	○	○	☐	-40	☐	
	L	Drugs	minimum possible	○	○	○	○	○	○	○	☐	0	☐	☐
			more than minimum	○	○	○	○	○	○	○	☐	-40	☐	
	M	Tobacco	didn't smoke	○	○	○	○	○	○	○	☐	0	☐	☐
			smoked	○	○	○	○	○	○	○	☐	-50	☐	

Weekly Weight Management Index (sum of items C+E+G+H+I) ☐

Overall Wellness Index (sums of all items) ☐

		OBJECTIVE		S	M	T	W	T	F	S	#	X	=	TOTAL
STRESS MANAGEMENT	A	Clarity and Personal Organization	clear & organized	◯	◯	◯	◯	◯	◯	◯		45		
			a bit disorganized	◯	◯	◯	◯	◯	◯	◯		30		
			poorly organized	◯	◯	◯	◯	◯	◯	◯		15		
	B	Attitude Control	positive attitude	◯	◯	◯	◯	◯	◯	◯		90		
			mostly positive	◯	◯	◯	◯	◯	◯	◯		60		
			negative attitude	◯	◯	◯	◯	◯	◯	◯		30		
	C	Conscious Relaxation	at least 5 minutes	◯	◯	◯	◯	◯	◯	◯		75		
			less than 5 minutes	◯	◯	◯	◯	◯	◯	◯		25		
PHYSICAL ACTIVITY	D	Full-Body Stretching	stretched	◯	◯	◯	◯	◯	◯	◯		60		
			didn't stretch	◯	◯	◯	◯	◯	◯	◯		20		
	E	Most Recent Aerobic Workout	this day	◯	◯	◯	◯	◯	◯	◯		120		
			the day before	◯	◯	◯	◯	◯	◯	◯		80		
			2 or more days prior	◯	◯	◯	◯	◯	◯	◯		40		
	F	Most Recent Body Toning Workout	this day	◯	◯	◯	◯	◯	◯	◯		30		
			1 or 2 days before	◯	◯	◯	◯	◯	◯	◯		20		
			3 or more days prior	◯	◯	◯	◯	◯	◯	◯		10		
NUTRITIONAL INTAKE	G	Amount of Food Eaten	moderate	◯	◯	◯	◯	◯	◯	◯		60		
			a bit too much	◯	◯	◯	◯	◯	◯	◯		40		
			excessive	◯	◯	◯	◯	◯	◯	◯		20		
	H	Intake of Unrefined Carbohydrates	high	◯	◯	◯	◯	◯	◯	◯		75		
			medium	◯	◯	◯	◯	◯	◯	◯		50		
			low	◯	◯	◯	◯	◯	◯	◯		25		
	I	Intake of Fats	low fat	◯	◯	◯	◯	◯	◯	◯		75		
			medium fat	◯	◯	◯	◯	◯	◯	◯		50		
			high fat	◯	◯	◯	◯	◯	◯	◯		25		
CHEMICAL INDEPENDENCE	J	Caffeine	1 cup or less	◯	◯	◯	◯	◯	◯	◯		0		
			2-3 cups	◯	◯	◯	◯	◯	◯	◯		-5		
			more than 3 cups	◯	◯	◯	◯	◯	◯	◯		-10		
	K	Alcohol	1 serving or less	◯	◯	◯	◯	◯	◯	◯		0		
			2 servings	◯	◯	◯	◯	◯	◯	◯		-10		
			3 or more servings	◯	◯	◯	◯	◯	◯	◯		-40		
	L	Drugs	minimum possible	◯	◯	◯	◯	◯	◯	◯		0		
			more than minimum	◯	◯	◯	◯	◯	◯	◯		-40		
	M	Tobacco	didn't smoke	◯	◯	◯	◯	◯	◯	◯		0		
			smoked	◯	◯	◯	◯	◯	◯	◯		-50		

Weekly Weight Management Index (sum of items C+E+G+H+I)

Overall Wellness Index (sums of all items)

DAILY PERFORMANCE RECORD – WEEK 4

		OBJECTIVE		S	M	T	W	T	F	S	#	X	=	TOTAL
STRESS MANAGEMENT	A	Clarity and Personal Organization	clear & organized									45		
			a bit disorganized									30		
			poorly organized									15		
	B	Attitude Control	positive attitude									90		
			mostly positive									60		
			negative attitude									30		
	C	Conscious Relaxation	at least 5 minutes									75		
			less than 5 minutes									25		
PHYSICAL ACTIVITY	D	Full-Body Stretching	stretched									60		
			didn't stretch									20		
	E	Most Recent Aerobic Workout	this day									120		
			the day before									80		
			2 or more days prior									40		
	F	Most Recent Body Toning Workout	this day									30		
			1 or 2 days before									20		
			3 or more days prior									10		
NUTRITIONAL INTAKE	G	Amount of Food Eaten	moderate									60		
			a bit too much									40		
			excessive									20		
	H	Intake of Unrefined Carbohydrates	high									75		
			medium									50		
			low									25		
	I	Intake of Fats	low fat									75		
			medium fat									50		
			high fat									25		
CHEMICAL INDEPENDENCE	J	Caffeine	1 cup or less									0		
			2-3 cups									-5		
			more than 3 cups									-10		
	K	Alcohol	1 serving or less									0		
			2 servings									-10		
			3 or more servings									-40		
	L	Drugs	minimum possible									0		
			more than minimum									-40		
	M	Tobacco	didn't smoke									0		
			smoked									-50		

Weekly Weight Management Index (sum of items C+E+G+H+I)	
Overall Wellness Index (sums of all items)	

		OBJECTIVE		S	M	T	W	T	F	S	#	X	=	TOTAL
STRESS MANAGEMENT	A	Clarity and Personal Organization	clear & organized	◯	◯	◯	◯	◯	◯	◯	☐	45	☐	☐
			a bit disorganized	◯	◯	◯	◯	◯	◯	◯		30		
			poorly organized	◯	◯	◯	◯	◯	◯	◯		15		
	B	Attitude Control	positive attitude	◯	◯	◯	◯	◯	◯	◯	☐	90	☐	☐
			mostly positive	◯	◯	◯	◯	◯	◯	◯		60		
			negative attitude	◯	◯	◯	◯	◯	◯	◯		30		
	C	Conscious Relaxation	at least 5 minutes	◯	◯	◯	◯	◯	◯	◯	☐	75	☐	☐
			less than 5 minutes	◯	◯	◯	◯	◯	◯	◯		25		
PHYSICAL ACTIVITY	D	Full-Body Stretching	stretched	◯	◯	◯	◯	◯	◯	◯	☐	60	☐	☐
			didn't stretch	◯	◯	◯	◯	◯	◯	◯		20		
	E	Most Recent Aerobic Workout	this day	◯	◯	◯	◯	◯	◯	◯	☐	120	☐	☐
			the day before	◯	◯	◯	◯	◯	◯	◯		80		
			2 or more days prior	◯	◯	◯	◯	◯	◯	◯		40		
	F	Most Recent Body Toning Workout	this day	◯	◯	◯	◯	◯	◯	◯	☐	30	☐	☐
			1 or 2 days before	◯	◯	◯	◯	◯	◯	◯		20		
			3 or more days prior	◯	◯	◯	◯	◯	◯	◯		10		
NUTRITIONAL INTAKE	G	Amount of Food Eaten	moderate	◯	◯	◯	◯	◯	◯	◯	☐	60	☐	☐
			a bit too much	◯	◯	◯	◯	◯	◯	◯		40		
			excessive	◯	◯	◯	◯	◯	◯	◯		20		
	H	Intake of Unrefined Carbohydrates	high	◯	◯	◯	◯	◯	◯	◯	☐	75	☐	☐
			medium	◯	◯	◯	◯	◯	◯	◯		50		
			low	◯	◯	◯	◯	◯	◯	◯		25		
	I	Intake of Fats	low fat	◯	◯	◯	◯	◯	◯	◯	☐	75	☐	☐
			medium fat	◯	◯	◯	◯	◯	◯	◯		50		
			high fat	◯	◯	◯	◯	◯	◯	◯		25		
CHEMICAL INDEPENDENCE	J	Caffeine	1 cup or less	◯	◯	◯	◯	◯	◯	◯	☐	0	☐	☐
			2-3 cups	◯	◯	◯	◯	◯	◯	◯		-5		
			more than 3 cups	◯	◯	◯	◯	◯	◯	◯		-10		
	K	Alcohol	1 serving or less	◯	◯	◯	◯	◯	◯	◯	☐	0	☐	☐
			2 servings	◯	◯	◯	◯	◯	◯	◯		-10		
			3 or more servings	◯	◯	◯	◯	◯	◯	◯		-40		
	L	Drugs	minimum possible	◯	◯	◯	◯	◯	◯	◯	☐	0	☐	☐
			more than minimum	◯	◯	◯	◯	◯	◯	◯		-40		
	M	Tobacco	didn't smoke	◯	◯	◯	◯	◯	◯	◯	☐	0	☐	☐
			smoked	◯	◯	◯	◯	◯	◯	◯		-50		

Weekly Weight Management Index (sum of items C+E+G+H+I) ☐

Overall Wellness Index (sums of all items) ☐

DAILY PERFORMANCE RECORD – WEEK 6

	OBJECTIVE		S	M	T	W	T	F	S	#	X	=	TOTAL
STRESS MANAGEMENT	**A** Clarity and Personal Organization	clear & organized									45		
		a bit disorganized									30		
		poorly organized									15		
	B Attitude Control	positive attitude									90		
		mostly positive									60		
		negative attitude									30		
	C Conscious Relaxation	at least 5 minutes									75		
		less than 5 minutes									25		
PHYSICAL ACTIVITY	**D** Full-Body Stretching	stretched									60		
		didn't stretch									20		
	E Most Recent Aerobic Workout	this day									120		
		the day before									80		
		2 or more days prior									40		
	F Most Recent Body Toning Workout	this day									30		
		1 or 2 days before									20		
		3 or more days prior									10		
NUTRITIONAL INTAKE	**G** Amount of Food Eaten	moderate									60		
		a bit too much									40		
		excessive									20		
	H Intake of Unrefined Carbohydrates	high									75		
		medium									50		
		low									25		
	I Intake of Fats	low fat									75		
		medium fat									50		
		high fat									25		
CHEMICAL INDEPENDENCE	**J** Caffeine	1 cup or less									0		
		2-3 cups									-5		
		more than 3 cups									-10		
	K Alcohol	1 serving or less									0		
		2 servings									-10		
		3 or more servings									-40		
	L Drugs	minimum possible									0		
		more than minimum									-40		
	M Tobacco	didn't smoke									0		
		smoked									-50		

Weekly Weight Management Index (sum of items C+E+G+H+I)

Overall Wellness Index (sums of all items)

After you have completed this six-week cycle, retake the Lifestyle Inventory, and establish your goals for the next six weeks.

WEIGHT CONTROL PROGRESS CHART

CHART THE POUNDS WHICH YOU ARE LOSING EACH WEEK

WEEK	DATE	WGT	1	2	3	4	5	6	7	8	9	10	11	12	13	14	15	16	17	18	19	20	21	22	23	24	25
1																											
2																											
3																											
4																											
5																											
6																											
7																											
8																											
9																											
10																											
11																											
12																											
13																											
14																											
15																											
16																											
17																											
18																											
19																											
20																											

RESTING HEART RATE PROGRESS CHART

CHART THE REDUCTIONS IN YOUR RESTING HEART RATE EACH WEEK

WEEK	DATE	RATE	1	2	3	4	5	6	7	8	9	10	11	12	13	14	15	16	17	18	19	20	21	22	23	24	25
1																											
2																											
3																											
4																											
5																											
6																											
7																											
8																											
9																											
10																											
11																											
12																											
13																											
14																											
15																											
16																											
17																											
18																											
19																											
20																											

LONG-TERM PROGRESS RECORD

Instructions: The Long-Term Progress Record provides you with a colorful display which enables you to see at a glance where your current living patterns are solidly supportive of your lasting well-being, and where they could use a bit of positive reinforcement. It also allows you to quickly recognize the progress you're making in the establishment of a well-balanced personal lifestyle for yourself.

To maintain this record, you'll need three different brightly colored pencils — red, yellow and green are ideal because of the powerful symbolic value which they already possess. Keep your Positive Lifestyle pens handy for ease of use whenever you need them.

At the end of each week, translate the Daily Performance Record weekly totals into their appropriate colors for entry here. Do this by referring to the "Mid-Range or Yellow Values" listed for each objective. When your weekly scores fall within these ranges, color the corresponding oval spaces yellow. When your scores are above the yellow range, color the ovals green. And when they fall below the yellow range, color those ovals red.

That's all there is to it. Simply update this visual record each week, and you'll always be in the perfect position to see exactly how you're doing across the entire array of key wellness factors. And best of all, it only takes a few moments for you to keep it up.

		Mid-Range or Yellow Values
A.	Goal Clarity	180-240
B.	Attitude Control	360-480
C.	Conscious Relaxation	275-375
D.	Stretching	220-300
E.	Aerobic Activity	480-600
F.	Body Toning	110-150
G.	Eating Independence	240-320
H.	Complex Carbohydrate	300-400
I.	Fat Intake	300-400
J.	Caffeine Independence	(35)-(15)
K.	Alcohol Independence	(40)-(20)
L.	Drug Independence	(40)
M.	Tobacco Independence	*
	Weight Management Index	1,535-2,135
	Positive Lifestyling Index	2,390-3,360

CYCLE 1 — Wk 1 2 3 4 5 6
CYCLE 2 — 1 2 3 4 5 6
CYCLE 3 — 1 2 3 4 5 6
CYCLE 4 — 1 2 3 4 5 6

* "0" equals green; any other score equals red.

DAILY CALORIE INTAKE CHART

Today's Date: _____

	Food Items	Amount	# Calories
B R E A K F A S T			
L U N C H			
D I N N E R			
S N A C K S			

Add up today's caloric intake: **Total number of calories consumed this day**		_____
Minus: **Approximate number of calories expended this day** (see page 46)		−_____
Equals: **Today's Calorie Surplus or (Calorie Deficit)**		=_____

Instructions: (Note–You may make as many copies of this particular form as you may need for your own personal use)
1. Using one copy of this form per day, record everything you eat–be sure to include quantities for all items.
2. Use the *Table of Food Composition* (page 41) to determine the number of calories represented by each food item.
3. Refer to the table on page 46 to approximate number of calories needed to sustain your level of activity on this day.
4. Subtract calories expended from total calories consumed to arrive at your calorie surplus or deficit for the day.

Keep the record for as many days as are required to develop what you feel is a representative sample of your eating patterns.

BODY TONING PROGRESS CHART

DATE:																		
Push-Ups																		
Hip Raises																		
Side Leg Lifts																		
Inner-Thigh Raise																		
Towel Stretch																		
Push & Pull																		
Neck Isometrics																		
Half Squats																		
Calf Raises																		
Full Leg & Buttock Tightening																		

Instructions: This form may help you to maintain a smooth progression in your body toning activities (you may make as many copies of this form as you need for your own personal use). To use it, make your entries for each workout in a single column, entering the date of the workout in the space provided at the top of the column.

The exercises on the upper half of the page correspond to the body toning exercises provided on pages 30 and 31. In the upper left part of the square, enter the number of times you perform the specified exercise during each set of repetitions. In the lower right part of the square enter the number of sets of repetitions you perform for the exercise.

Alternatively, the bottom part of the page provides a means of keeping track of your progress if you are using exercise machines or free weights for body toning. In this case, enter in the upper half of the square the number of repetitions you perform of each exercise, and, in the lower half, the amount of weight or resistance you are using.

SUBSTANCE USAGE RECORD

Date	Time	Substance	Amount	Circumstances, effects, other observations

Instructions: Use this form as an aid in observing your usage of any substance upon which you now have a dependence, or upon which you feel you could conceivably develop a dependence. You may make copies of this form for your own use.

THE QUALITIES OF WELLNESS

MORE WELL		LESS WELL
Strengthened, circulates more blood per beat, permits lower resting heart rate.	**Your Heart**	Weakened, circulates less blood per beat, requires higher resting heart rate.
Larger, more elastic, less obstructed with fat, freer circulation, lower blood pressure.	**Your Blood Vessels**	Constricted, inelastic, clogged with excess fat, reduced circulation, elevated blood pressure.
Decreased cholesterol (fat), triglycerides, blood sugar, insulin, adrenalin, clotting.	**Your Blood**	Increased cholesterol (fat), triglycerides, blood sugar, insulin, adrenalin, clotting.
Expanded capacity for oxygen absorption and waste expulsion.	**Your Lungs**	Restricted capacity for oxygen absorption and waste expulsion.
Generally elevated, more calories consumed in all activities, promotes leanness.	**Your Metabolic Rate**	Generally suppressed, fewer calories consumed per activity, tends to accumulate more fat.
Lean, with proportionally more muscle and bone.	**Your Body Composition**	Fat, with proportionally less muscle and bone.
Stronger, more dense and resilient.	**Your Bones**	Weaker, more porous and brittle.
Capable of a wide range of fluid motion.	**Your Joints**	Stiff, restricted, sometimes painful motion.
Stronger, more firm, defined and efficient, tending to burn more calories.	**Your Muscles**	Weaker, less toned and efficient, tending to burn fewer calories, less sensitive to insulin.
Alert, more clear and concentrated, less boredom and fatigue.	**Your Mental Functioning**	Dull, worried and distracted, more boredom and fatigue.
More patient, tolerant, relaxed and enthusiastic.	**Your Emotions**	Impatient, critical, tense and depressed.
Decreased risk due to healthier heart, lungs, blood vessels, liver, bones, muscle and body composition.	**Your Risk of Illness**	Increased risk of diseases of heart, lungs, blood vessels and liver; of diabetes, stroke, accidents and broken bones.
More active, generating greater vitality and endurance, tending toward health.	**Your Quality Of Life**	Inactive, generating less vitality and endurance, tending toward illness.
Possible extension beyond the average.	**Your Lifespan**	Possible reduction below the average.
More confident, with positive appreciation of self.	**Your Self-Concept**	Less certain, more doubtful and self-conscious.

Enjoy the many lasting benefits of living a life of health, fitness and well-being.

BIBLIOGRAPHY

Stress Management

Coping With Stress, Donald Meichenbaum (Century, UK, 1983).

Executive Health, Phillip Goldberg (McGraw Hill, 1978).

Executive Stress, Ari Kiev (AMACON, New York, 1980).

From Burnout To Balance, Dennis T. Jaffe and Cynthia D. Scott (McGraw-Hill, New York, 1984).

Happiness, Bloomfield and Kory (Simon & Schuster, New York, 1976).

Management of Stress: Using TM at Work, David R. Frew (Nelson-Hall, Chicago, 1977).

Managing Stress: Before It Manages You, Steinmetz, Blankenship, Brown, Hall and Miller (Bull Publishing Company, 1980).

Massage Book, The, George Downing (Random House, New York, 1972).

Mind As Healer, Mind As Slayer, K. Pelletier (Delacore Press, 1976).

New Mind, New Body, Barbara Brown (Harper & Row, New York, 1974).

Progressive Relaxation, Edmond Jacobson (University of Chicago Press, 1938).

Psychology of Consciousness, The, Robert Ornstein (Freeman, San Francisco, 1972).

Relax, White and Fadiman, eds. (Confucian Press, New York, 1976).

Relaxation and Stress Reduction Workbook, The, Davis, Eshelman, Mckay (New Harbinger, Oakland, 1982).

Relaxation Response, The, Herbert Benson (Morrow, New York, 1975).

Stress And The Manager: Making It Work For You, K. Albrecht (Prentice-Hall, Englewood Cliffs, NJ, 1979).

Stress Without Distress, Hans Selye (Lippincott, 1974).

TM and Business, Jay B. Marcus (McGraw-Hill, New York, 1978).

TM Program: The Way to Fulfillment, The, Philip Goldberg (Holt, Rinehart & Winston, New York, 1976).

Type A Behavior and Your Heart, Meyer Friedman and Ray Rosenman (Fawcett, New York, 1974).

You Must Relax, Edmond Jacobson (McGraw-Hill, New York, 1957).

Exercise

Aerobics for Women, M. Cooper and K. Cooper (Bantam Books, New York, 1979).

Aerobics Program for Total Well-Being, The, Kenneth Cooper (Evans & Co., New York, 1982).

Beauty of Running, The, G. Barron, (Harcourt, Brace, Jovanovich, New York, 1980).

Beyond Diet: Exercise Your Way To Fitness and Heart Health, Lenore Zohman. Pamphlet, free from Mazola Nutrition Information Service; Dept. ZD-NYT, Box 307, Coventry, CT 06238.

Bike Tripping, Tom Cuthbertson (Ten Speed Press, Berkeley, CA, 1972).

Complete Book of Running, The, James Fixx (Random House, New York, 1977).

Dr. Marchetti's Walking Book, A. Marchetti (Stein and Day, 1980).

Dr. Sheehan On Running, George Sheehan, M.D. (Bantam Books, New York, 1978).

Exercise And Your Heart, # 555K, Consumer Information Center, Box 3D, Pueblo, CO 81009.

Exercise in the Office, Robert R. Spackman (Southern Illinois University Press, Carbondale, IL, 1968).

Fitness On The Road; Where To Stay To Stay Fit, John Winsor (Shelter Publications, Bolinas, CA, 1986).

Galloway's Book On Running, Jeff Galloway (Shelter Publications, Bolinas, CA, 1984).

Introduction to Yoga, Richard Hittleman (Bantam Books, New York, 1969)

Low Stress Fitness—An Easy Does It Exercise Plan For Any Age, Millie Brown (HP Books, Tucson, AZ, 1985).

Miracle of Rebound Exercise, The, Albert E. Carter (Snohomish Publishing Co., 1979).

New Aerobics, The, Kenneth Cooper (Evans & Co., New York, 1970).

Perfect Exercise, The, Curtis Mitchell (Simon & Schuster, New York, 1976).

Royal Canadian Air Force Exercise Plans For Physical Fitness, (Pocket Books, New York, 1972).

Running For Health and Beauty: A Complete Guide For Women, Kathryn Lance (Bobbs-Merrill, New York, 1977).

Running Free, Joan Ullyot, M.D. (Putnam & Sons, New York, 1982).

Stretching, Bob Anderson (Shelter Publications, Bolinas, CA 1980).

Nutrition

Athlete's Kitchen, The, Nancy Clar (C.B.I., Boston, 1981).

Diet and Nutrition, R. Ballantine (Himalayan International Institute, 1978).

Diet for a Small Planet, Frances Moore Lappé (Ballantine Books, New York, 1971).

Eater's Guide, The, Candy Cumming and Vicky Newman (Prentice-Hall, 1981).

Eat To Win; The Sports Nutrition Bible, Robert Haas (Tawson Associates, New York, 1983).

Live Longer Now, Leonard Hofer and Nathan Pritikin (Grosset & Dunlap, 1977).

Nutrition Almanac, Nutrition Search, Inc. (McGraw-Hill, 1979).

Oat Fiber, The Quaker Oats Company, 231 S. Green Street, Chicago, IL 60687

Orthomolecular Psychiatry, Linus Pauling (The Huxley Institute, New York).

Plant Fiber In Foods ($10—Order from HCF Diabetes Foundation, P.O. Box 22124, Lexington, KY 40522).

Psychodietetics: Food as the Key to Emotional Health, Cheraskin, Ringsdorf and Brecher (Stein & Day, New York, 1974).

Sugar Blues, William Dufty (Warner, New York, 1976).

Low Salt Cooking

Cooking Without Your Salt Shaker, American Heart Association (available through local chapters).

Craig Claiborne's Gourmet Diet, Craig Claiborne (Times Books, New York, 1980).

Good Age Cookbook, The, Jan Harlow, Irene Liggett and Evelyn Madel (Houghton-Mifflin, Boston, 1979).

Gourmet Cooking Without Salt, Eleanor P. Brenner (Doubleday, New York, 1981).

Living With High Blood Pressure—The Hypertension Diet Cookbook, Joyce Daly, Margie and Dr. James C. Hunt (Chilton Press, Radnor, PA, 1979).

Secrets of Salt Free Cooking, The, Jeanne Jones (Scribner's, 1979).

Weight Control

Act Thin, Stay Thin, Richard Stuart, Ph.D. (W.W. Norton, New York, 1978).

Diet Free!, Charles Kuntzleman, Ph.D. (Rodale, Emmaus, PA, 1982).

Dr. Anderson's Life-Saving Diet, Dr. James Anderson (Body Press, 1986).

Fit or Fat, Covert Bailey (Houghton Mifflin, 1977).

Eating Is Okay, Dr. Henry A. Jordan, Leonard S. Levitz, Ph.D. and Gordon M. Kimbrell, Ph.D. (Signet, New York, 1976)

How Mother's And Others Stay Slim, Lawrence Holt (California Health Publications, 1981).

How To Eat Like a Thin Person, Dusky, Lorraine, and Dr. J.J. Leady (Simon and Schuster, New York, 1982).

Permanent Weight Control, Kathryn Mahoney and Michael J. Mahoney, Ph.D. (W.W. Norton, New York, 1976).

Successful Dieting Tips, Bruce Lansky (Meadowbrook Press, Deephaven, MN, 1981)

Overall Wellness

American Way of Life Need Not Be Hazardous To Your Health, The, John W. Farquhar, M.D. (Norton, New York, 1978).

Complete Manual of Fitness and Well-Being, The, Robert Arnot (Viking Penguin, New York, 1984).

High-Energy Factor, The, Bernard Gutin with Gail Kessler (Random House, New York, 1983).

Hope Healthletter, International Health Awareness Center, 157 S. Kalamazoo Mall, Kalamazoo, MI 49007

Looking Great, Staying Young, Dick Clark (Bobbs-Merrill, Indianapolis, 1980).

Many-Dimensional Man, Jay Ogilvy (Harper & Row, New York, 1981).

New York Times Guide To Personal Health, The, Jane Brody (Times Books, New York, 1982).

Pathfinders, Gail Sheehy (Morrow, 1981).

Taking Charge of Your Weight and Well-Being, J.D. Nash & L.O. Orminston (Bull Publishing, Palo Alto, CA, 1978).

Well Body Book, The, M. Samuels and H. Bennett (Random House, New York, 1973).

Wellness Workbook, The, Regina Sara Ryan and John W. Travis, M.D. (Ten Speed Press, Berkeley, CA, 1981).

Dependencies

Cocaine—Seduction and Solution, Nannette Stone, Marlene Fromme, Daniel Kagan (Clarkson N. Polter, New York, 1984).

Dealing With Drink, Ian Davies and Duncan Raistrick (State Mutual Books, 1981).

Drugs In America: A Social History 1800-1980, H. Wayne Morgan (Syracuse University Press, 1981).

Facts About Drug Abuse, The, The Drug Abuse Council (Macmillan, New York, 1980).

How To Straighten Up Your Act and Keep The Money In The Country, Skip Haynes (Ursus Press, San Diego, 1985).

If Your Child Is Drinking, Nancy Hyden Woodward (Putnam, New York, 1981).

Kids & Drugs: A Parents' Handbook of Drug Abuse Prevention and Treatment, Jason D. Baron, M.D. (Putnam, New York, 1983).

Not My Kid; A Parent's Guide To Kids and Drugs, Beth Polson and Miller Newton (Arbor House, New York, 1984).

Underground Empire, James Mills (Doubleday, New York, 1986).

Exercise For The Elderly

Aging and Exercise, Dr. Everett L. Smith and Dr. Karl Stoedefalke ($4—Order from Dr. Smith, Department of Preventive Medicine, University of Wisconsin, 504 Walnut, Madison, WI 53706).

Be Alive as Long as You Live, ($10.95—Order from Preventicare Publications, 106 Brooks Street, Charleston, WV 25301).

Fitness, Vitality, and You, Dr. Robert E. Wear ($5—Order from Lionel E. Mayrand, Jr., Gerontology Department, New England Center for Continuing Education, University of New Hampshire, Durham, NH 03824).

Specialized Reading

A Good Age, Alex Comfort (Crown, 1978).

Book of Ages, The, Desmond Morris (Viking Penguin, New York, 1983).

Complete Guide to Symptoms, Illness & Surgery, H. Winter Griffith, M.D. (HP Books, Tucson, AZ, 1985).

Coping With Job Stress, H.M. Greenberg (Prentice-Hall, Englewood Cliffs, NJ, 1980).

Drugs—Complete Guide to Prescription & Non-Prescription, H. Winter Griffith, M.D. (HP Books, Tucson, AZ, Revised 1985).

Executive Health, P. Goldberg (McGraw-Hill, New York, 1978).

Guidelines for Graded Exercise Testing and Exercise Prescription (2nd edition), American College of Sports Medicine (Lea & Frebiger, Philadelphia, PA, 1980).

Health Promotion In The Workplace, Michael P. O'Donnell, Thomas Ainsworth, M.D., Editors (John Wiley & Sons, New York, 1984).

Healthy People: The Surgeon General's Report On Health Promotion and Disease Prevention, Department of Health, Education and Welfare (U.S. Government Printing Office, Washington, DC, 1979).

Inner Game of Tennis, The, W. Timothy Gallwey (Random House, New York, 1974).

Men At Midlife, Michael P. Farrell and Stanley D. Rosenberg (Auburn House, Boston, 1981).

Over The Hill, But Not Out To Lunch! Over 40 and Cookin', Ed LLoyd Kahn, Jr. (Shelter, Bolina, CA, 1986).

Power of Positive Thinking, Norman Vincent Peale (Fawcett, New York, 1978).

Pregnant & Beautiful—How to Eat Right, Stay Fit and Look Great, Lindsay R. Curtis, M.D., Cynthia Hazeltine, R.D., and Judith Rasband, M.S. (HP Books, Tucson, AZ, 1985).

Quaker Oats Company Newsletter (Free Oat Fiber Materials, 13-part Healthy Eating Recipes series, Nutritive Values Charts), Send request on a postcard to: Oat Fiber, The Quaker Oats Company, 231 S. Green Street, Chicago, IL 60607.

Richard's Bicycle Book, Richard Ballantine (Ballantine Books, Westminster, MD, 1972).

Seeing Yourself See—Eye Exercises For Total Vision, Jim Jackson (Saturday Review Press/Dutton, New York, 1975).

Self-Hypnotism: The Technique and its Use in Daily Living, L. Lecron (Prentice-Hall, Englewood Cliffs, NJ, 1964).

Total Nutrition During Pregnancy, Betty Kamen, Ph.D. and Si Kamen (Keats Publishing, New Canaan, CT, 1981).

What Color Is Your Parachute? (Job Hunter's Manual), Richard Bolles (Ten Speed Press, Berkeley, CA, 1980).

Women Coming Of Age, Jane Fonda (Simon & Schuster, New York, 1984).